DO YOU THINK I NEED TO WEAR BOOBS WITH THIS DRESS?

WESTCOM PRESS
Washington DC

DO YOU THINK I NEED TO WEAR BOOBS WITH THIS DRESS?

Redesigning life after breast cancer

LYNNE HANSON

Do You Think I Need to Wear Boobs with This Dress?
by Lynne Hanson

Copyright © 2013 Lynne Hanson

www.doineedboobs.org

Published by: Westcom Press
            2101 N Street, NW, Suite T-1
            Washington, DC 20037

            westcom.press@mac.com

ISBN - 978-1-938620-01-0

Library of Congress Control Number: 2012950282

Editor: Melanie Mallon

Cover art and design: Lynne Hanson and Chris Flynn

A portion of the proceeds from this book will be donated to organizations fighting to find the cure for breast cancer.

Printed in the United States of America
18 17 16 15 14 13 12   1 2 3 4 5

*To all the women dealing with the emotional
and physical scars of breast cancer
and to those who love them*

Contents

Prologue .... *xi*

1. I Always Wanted to Have Monica Silverman's Body..... 1
2. Zipper Number One 5
3. Unzipped 15
4. Mountain or Molehill 23
5. Decorating 101 27
6. Just Another Zipper 33
7. Pistachios in the Dark 39
8. Waking My Inner Dolly Parton 45
9. Inside Out 51
10. Farewell to Thee, Dolly Parton 57
11. Life Lopsided... 61
12. The Rise of Annie Flats 69
13. Strength in Numbers 75
14. Mona Soup and Matzo Ball Soup 79
15. Multiple Personalities 83
16. The 9/11 Snowball...87
17. Moving On 91
18. 5:30 p.m., Friday, January 17, 2003......................97
19. Care Bears and Casserole......................................105

20. Just Close Your Eyes, Grit Your Teeth, and Do It 111

21. Where in the World Is Chelsea Hanson? 121

22. Is It My Turn? 123

23. Hello Good-bye 127

24. OMG, the Kentucky Derby! 131

25. Rowena 135

26. Signs 139

27. The Next Leap..145

28. Women without Partners 151

29. Patience, Prudence...157

30. Vamoose 163

31. With a Little Help from the Pros................................167

32. Annie's Debut 173

33. Annie Goes to Bloomingdale's 179

34. Standing Naked in Front of Class..............................185

35. A Perfect Tee 193

36. The Real Reveal..197

37. Aw, It's Your First Bra . . . Again................................201

38. Do You Think I Need to Wear Boobs
    with This Dress? 211

39. Mom, You're Migrating...217

40. Full Circle 225

Acknowledgments *233*

Prologue

$\mathcal{I}$ needed to make a dress form that was more like me. My chest was deformed from my mastectomies, and it was important to replicate the changes in my body. I had purchased a dress form that had small breasts, but as I tried on clothes, then put them on the form, I saw that our shapes were massively different. Building up the chest area by wrapping fabric around the breasts did not work. It was clear that I had to remove, not build up. There was no way I could really get to the bottom of my fit problem with a form that was not accurate.

I removed the outer fabric of the dress form, not sure what I would find underneath. Layers and layers of fabric came off until I finally reached a rough fiberglass frame. I got out all the saws I had in my immense collection. Through the years, I had acquired every type of cutting device in existence, from an assortment of X-acto knives that filled a small antique wooden box to the huge radial arm saw tucked away in the corner of my garage.

I started with a mat cutter and ended up using a sleek triangular handsaw that my sister Jamie had given me. It was effortless to saw away the tiny breasts. They melted away like butter. It felt wonderful. Cathartic. The saw and I were one, as shards of fiberglass flew around me.

But the form was still not right.

I measured the rib cage area, which I had not touched. The entire chest area around the missing breasts was not right. I needed to cut away more. Again and again, I sawed away, measuring the proportions against mine and needing to remove even more. How could that be? The surgeon had taken away my breasts, not my entire body. The scars extended only across my chest, not down the rib cage. How big could my mosquito-size breasts have really been?

It was not until most of the chest and rib cage area was gone that I finally got the right proportions. I was shocked. The massive hole in the form went vertically from just below the collar bone, almost to the waist, and horizontally all the way across to under the arms. All this was taken away from my body, I thought. This was what was taken from me.

I was beginning to understand why women who have had mastectomies need to grieve. We have lost a lot. Not only part of what defines our femininity, but a good chunk of ourselves. Although a breast is not a limb, it is not a mole either. Our bodies have been violated, and they need to heal, which takes time, courage, and support. To throw two plastic bags they call implants into our bodies does not truly fill the gaping hole left by what we have lost.

I needed to help other women and myself. I had not understood until now. This was my purpose in life.

Chapter One

I Always Wanted to Have Monica Silverman's Body

I grew up in the fifties and sixties, in suburban Maryland, just outside DC. My neighborhood was filled with the brainpower of government intellectuals and international dignitaries.

I was the middle child. Not academic, like the rest of my family, but the imaginative one. I was always working on something, my drawers filled with everything from architectural drawings to sketches of clothing ensembles. Creative and stubborn, I was not happy with my given name, so in second grade, I asked my mother to please inform my teacher that, from now on, I was to be called Tzuzi, my version of Suzanne, my middle name. Lynne was far too boring for the likes of me. As the years progressed, my collection of names grew to include Dimps (for my dimples); Umpossible, because my parents always told me I was "umpossible," as in stubborn; and Lisa, my persona from

1

design school in New York City (although my roommate called me Lynnard). I was still Lisa when I transferred to San Diego, where I met my husband, Alan. Lisa stuck around for just a short time, but Lynnard has stuck to this day.

My older sister, Jamie, whom I hated and worshipped at the same time, loved to argue with people (she ended up in law school) and would scare away my friends. But if she told me that the sky was green, I would believe her and defend to my death that the sky was green. My younger sister, Lauren, spent her time making hovercrafts out of vacuum motors and contemplating how to better the world. She was her own person and had no interest in becoming a "Jamie groupie."

Life was good, except for my never-ending desire to have Monica Silverman's body. She was thin and beautiful, every feature dainty and perfect. Always the popular one, she was sophisticated, having lived in France for two years. In high school she was a pom pom girl and one of the smart girls. Education and brains were valued at our school; it was cool to be smart. I was not in the "in crowd." At school I kept to myself, and the minute classes let out, I was off to my horses or swim team practice, following in Jamie's footsteps. I had developed hips and curves in the era of Twiggy. I wanted so badly to be like Monica.

But doesn't everyone have body issues?

Breasts were not one of mine. My butt and thighs were my issue. I always felt like people looked at me and thought, "There goes thunder thighs," but my breasts and flat tummy were my source of pride. Even after nursing two children, I loved my breasts. Sure, they could have used a little lift, but they were still great. I was not large. In college I was a AA, and while pregnant and nursing, I made a B cup, but usually I was an A/A-plus—not big, but beautiful. They were symmetrical, something I discovered was rare among us natural-chested women (and I have since learned that the "enhanced" women have issues with symmetry too).

Chapter Two

Zipper Number One

I started getting mammograms every year at age thirty-two, after my mother was diagnosed with breast cancer. Breast cancer was prevalent in my extended family as well, among the many wonderful ailments that come with being of Eastern European Jewish descent, so I was very conscious of my risk. My grandparents had immigrated from Eastern Europe to New York City's impoverished but flavorful Lower East Side. In the forties my parents, Nee and Sid, left the comfort of NYC and boldly went where no relative had gone before: Washington, DC. It was a revolt of epic proportions to leave New York, and we heard about it constantly from our extended family.

The only problem with my breasts was trying to fit them in the mammography machine. The mammogram was always a fun process. I am only five-foot four, so I had to stand precariously on my toes to reach the machine, trying to keep my balance while my tiny breasts were flattened out between two sheets of Plexiglas.

This device was definitely invented by a man. So why hasn't a man come up with another product, less barbaric than one that puts forty pounds of pressure on the one part of a woman's body that men so cherish? And even more puzzling, why hasn't a woman come up with something better?

"Hi, sweetie," the nurse would chime. "Now, this isn't going to hurt a bit." Really. Did she honestly think I would buy that? I have never understood why other women lie to us like this. Of course it's going to hurt! *You have breasts too. You know it's going to hurt.*

So, it was not a total surprise when, in late spring 1990, just before my fortieth birthday, the radiologist found a suspicious cloudy area in my left breast. The doctor ordered an ultrasound, but the results were inconclusive. I was surprisingly calm when he then suggested a lumpectomy. He explained that I could go without one and have another ultrasound at a later date, but I was not comfortable with that. Not with my family history. A lumpectomy was the most drastic of my options, but I did not want to leave any doubt as to what this lump was. I was young—far too young to have cancer—so I was not worried. I just wanted to make sure.

I was scheduled for a very early morning outpatient surgery with general anesthesia. Alan, my husband of seventeen years, was at my side. We had been through a lot together, surviving moves all along the West Coast, trying to avoid the "establishment" lifestyle only to end up in Seattle, sucked into the lavish perks of corporate and suburban life. Until now, our family's health concerns had revolved around our daughters—our youngest, Chelsea, had asthma, and her sister, Braiden, had suffered many illnesses and injuries, including chronic life-threatening food allergies.

We had made arrangements for the girls, now ten and eight, to go to friends' houses after school. Braiden would miss her ice-skating lessons, and Chelsea her basketball practice, but we did not tell them much, just that I had to have a medical procedure and would be home later. After all, this was just a precautionary procedure that would simply confirm that all was well.

As we silently waited for a nurse to summoned us, Alan read a magazine, and I read Alan. I studied his round face, his small ski jump nose scrunched over his graying mustache. His black hair had more gray in it too and was starting to thin. Alan's father was Norwegian, his mother Pacific Northwest Native American (Okanogan), which made for an interesting blend: he was a dark-eyed, curly-haired, small but stocky, Asian-looking Viking. Yes, our kids are Native American, Norwegian Jews.

When I'd first starting dating Alan, back in college, I'd called my mom to tell her. We had a regular dialogue that we always joked about whenever I dated someone new.

"Hi, Mom. I met someone."

"Oh, is he?" Meaning, "Is he Jewish?" She knew that I rarely dated anyone Jewish, so she always said it in an "I already know the answer and I'm very disappointed" way.

"No, he's not," I would always answer. But this time I'd added, "But he is Native American."

"Oh, wow! That's just as good!" she had exclaimed. "They've been persecuted too, so he knows what it's like and can understand."

Now, in the waiting room, I chuckled, and Alan glanced up to see me staring at him. "What?" he asked, but before I could answer, my name was called.

I was taken to a private room and asked to change into every patient's favorite garment—the infamous blue-and-white patterned examination gown. I didn't understand why this garment was open in the back when they have to get to the boob in the front. Maybe the medical world liked to make us so uncomfortable that we wouldn't worry about the surgery. It never occurred to me that I was wearing it wrong.

"Hey darling," the pudgy, fifties-something technician said, grinning. One of my pet peeves is a stranger calling me endearing names like darling. *I don't know you, and I'm not your darling.*

"Sweetie," she continued condescendingly, "you need to change your dressing gown so that it opens in the front."

Oh boy. Not only would I have the humiliation of the mastectomy machine, but I had to remove my dressing gown in front of the uber-cheery technician. Why is it called a dressing gown anyway? Are we dressing up or down?

The first order of business was for the technicians to locate the lump. As I stood on my tiptoes, hanging onto the mammography machine, my breast clamped between the Plexiglas sheets, they would first locate the suspicious area, then, while I was fully awake, one would stick a wire into my breast to pinpoint it exactly for the surgery. I do not like needles, so usually when I get a shot, I look away and pinch my neck to distract myself from the needle prick. I did that, although I cannot tell you how in the world I managed while hanging on to that machine, and surprisingly, it did not hurt when they stuck the wire into my skin.

They let me out of the torture machine, and I stood there, at first just impressed with the proficiency of the technician but then gradually wondering how I would know if she got the right area. Then it hit me. There was a wire sticking out of my breast. *There's a wire sticking out of my breast!* The room started swirling, and I began to slump to the floor. The technicians caught me and gently sat me in a nearby chair. I guess this happens all the time; there was another wooden chair alongside me, ready to catch the next patient.

"Okay, honey, you just sit yourself down here." Nurse Sweetcakes's dyed brownish hair brushed across my shoulder. It was a color that said, I am not red, I am not brown, I am not gray, I am not anything. I hate that color.

It is one of the stranger sights to look down and see a wire protruding from one's breast. No blood, no redness, no nothing—just a long straight wire sticking out about six inches. It was dark and made from a few thin wires twisted together, like trash bag twisty ties. Not pretty. A colorful one might have been nicer. You could pick your own color, just as you can pick your cast color when you break an arm. I would have gone for some loud, happy color, or maybe a few different colors to make an interesting design in the twist.

I sat on the chair for a while, my head between my legs, trying not to pass out or throw up. I am not good with nausea; I hardly ever throw up, and I am a real weenie about it. Never fainted either, and I was not about to start. I was determined to be strong, so I gathered myself together and returned to my room in a wheelchair to wait for the lumpectomy.

Alan was waiting in the room, his dark eyes fixated on a TV screen bigger than we had at home. He looked like he was in heaven. I doubt he saw the wire, which was sticking out between the ties of my blue-and-white gown. Sexy.

"Okay, sweetie, we'll just leave you here until you feel better." My not-so-favorite nurse left us alone. "What are you watching?" I asked Alan. By now the adrenaline rush had worn off and I was exhausted.

"*Judge Judy.*"

"Who's Judge Judy?"

"Don't know, but she's mean."

He was not really watching it, though, and neither was I. The noise of the TV allowed us to be left to our own thoughts and fears, pondering the uncertain future in solitude. The idea that something might be wrong seemed unimaginable. I was way too young.

"What are you drinking?" I asked after some time.

"I think they meant it to be coffee."

"Oh."

We returned to our silence. He was right. Judge Judy was mean.

After what seemed an eternity, a teenage aide, probably checking out her nursing career options, came to take me into surgery.

"Enjoy *Judge Judy.*"

Alan gave me a kiss and a loving but worried nod. I recalled the time when he'd had surgery on his back. As they'd wheeled him away, he had refused to give up his bottle-thick glasses, as if to say, "If I can't see, I'm gone."

I felt like everyone we passed along the long and barren hallways was staring at my wire. I did not want to look at anyone and hated staring up at the ceiling while lying on my gurney. My eyes glazed over, and I tried to ignore my discomfort and let my mind wander.

The aide took me to the prep room, a sterile room with tile walls and the background hum of doctors, nurses, and medical equipment in use. I was lined up alongside other ladies on gurneys, all of us fully conscious, awaiting unknown diagnoses and fates. Lambs lined up for the slaughter. We did not talk. We were too far away from each other to have a conversation, much less an intimate one about breasts and wires.

We were all given IVs and hair caps to go with our beautiful gowns. The nurses and aides were great, checking on us and making sure we were warm and as comfortable as possible. Every time we were moved, our wristbands were checked to make sure we were who we needed to be. That gave me a small inkling of reassurance that a lump and my wire would be the only things removed from my body.

"Hey, cookie." Nurse Sweetcakes put a warm blanket over me and gave me a gentle pat on my thigh. I could smell her Juicy Fruit gum. "You just wait here. Let us know if you need anything, and we'll be back to get you as soon as the doctor is ready."

When it was my turn, I was wheeled into a surgery room, which was nothing like the rooms on *Grey's Anatomy* or *ER*. It was tiny, with few machines and many people, and it was colder than Alaska (my kind of weather!). My surgeon, Dr. Williams, and I had already bonded over tales of the great outdoors, comparing skiing and white-water-rafting trips in Jackson Hole, Wyoming, and Utah. I hear that lots of women develop crushes on their doctors, and I was no exception. He was handsome, compassionate, and about to cut my breast open. How romantic.

"Ready?" he asked me. I could not see his thick brown hair or sparkly eyes under his cap and mask.

"Sure, let's do it."

And the next thing I knew, I was opening my eyes in the recovery room to a whopper of a headache. I groaned, "Where's Alan?" At least I remembered his name. Nurse Sweetcakes noticed me talking to myself.

"He's waiting for you in your room, darling, watching TV."

At that point, I guess she could call me darling. She could call me anything she wanted.

They rolled me up to my room, where Alan and I watched more TV and waited for the anesthesia to wear off. I had a huge bandage across my chest. The anesthesia had made me incredibly nauseated, and the bedpan became my new best friend. Alan had been on ski patrol for many years and had seen many injuries, so blood and vomit did not faze him. He just went with the flow. They discharged me within a few hours of my procedure, after I had regained more consciousness and stopped throwing up for an hour.

My scar was about four inches long and ran across the top portion of my breast. I wondered why Dr. Williams had chosen to put the scar there, where it would be easy to see when I wore low-cut clothing. Maybe he loved me so much that he did not want me to share my breasts with others. It did not occur to me at the time that it made the most sense to cut there, because it was the most direct way to the lump. Dr. Williams was not a plastic surgeon. He was just doing his job.

After a few weeks, the swelling went down, and there was a small dent in the breast just below the slightly raised red scar, which sort of looked like a large zipper. I did not see the need to make such a big statement, but there it was, and I would live with it. The assurance that there was no cancer was by far worth the dent and scar on my perfect breasts.

Chapter Three

Unzipped

I moved on from the surgery and was back to my world, without a thought that the outcome could be cancer. My parents came to visit, and as always, we had a great time together. They were the best grandparents anyone could ask for, and Alan and my father had an extremely close bond, in part because they shared many interests and in part because Alan was not very close to his parents, so my father had become Alan's father.

My parents had recently retired from their careers in DC, my father with the Pentagon (to this day we are not sure what he did) and my mother, former supervisor for special education in the prestigious Montgomery County School District in Maryland. They had moved to San Diego, where my father kept busy with tennis and my mother with her belly dancing and TV production classes. Mom even started a career in TV news broadcasting, and eventually won two Emmys for her work coproducing documentaries.

It was a long weekend, and Alan had gone mountain climbing with his cousin Jon in the nearby Cascades. Jon was one of the few people I felt comfortable letting Alan climb with as Jon was an even more accomplished climber, which was saying a lot considering Alan's outdoor obsessions— skiing, mountain climbing, fly-fishing, you name it. With other climbing buddies, Alan would climb a mountain carrying his skis, then ski down it. When we'd lived in Portland, Oregon, one of his friends had commented, after a pre-dawn climb of Mt. Hood, "Having fun with Alan means it has to hurt."

Skiing was an activity he shared with the girls, too. In fact, Braiden and Chelsea were skiing before they could walk. At fifteen months, Braiden would cheer with delight as Alan skied down a hill with her on his shoulders. He would go over small jumps and her face would light up while mine went gray with fear.

In Seattle, he had become obsessed with fly-fishing, and he, Braiden, and Chelsea would religiously watch the TV show *Fishing the West* with their official *Fishing the West* baseball hats firmly on their heads. The three of them had their own fly-tying equipment and loved to experiment with the colorful threads and feathers that Alan had collected. He would take them out on our drift boat, a specialized boat used for floating down rivers while fishing. I would drive them to a launching point and they, along with our dog, Beans, would climb into the boat and drift off for me to pick them up farther downstream. It was always catch and release, and the serenity of the river, forests, and mountains was their bonding time.

So while Alan and Jon were away that Friday, the rest of us headed to the mall. My parents were clotheshorses—my debonair father loved to wear the latest fashion, and my mother loved to buy anything on sale.

"Here, you'll love this." I hated when my mother said this. How did she know what I would love? She shoved the shirt within inches of my face. She was always buying me clothes on sale that I did not want. They looked like they were the last of the sale rack. "And I got it on sale."

"Thanks, but it's really not me," I told her, trying not to hurt her feelings.

"No, it's you. It's exactly what you wear." Her slightly antiqued face was more determined than ever. She eyed my baggy sweats and oversized T-shirt. "And you don't have to iron it."

She had me there. I hated ironing and avoided it like the plague. But I hated this shirt too. It was almost as big as a painter's smock, with pale pink and white pinstripes. I never wore pink. The pocket on the left side had an embroidered design on it, like a family crest, but I don't think it meant anything. Another clothing company trying to create a snobby image.

I had designed clothes for companies such as Pendleton Woolen Mills and White Stag, yet I was like the cobbler who had holes in her shoes. Though always aware of the latest fashions, and sometimes willing to try them, I would inevitably return to my comfort zone of jeans, sweats, and tees. After all, my life consisted of carpools and grocery stores, and I was not concerned with how the skating moms and the grocery checkout clerks saw me. I wanted to spend my time creating.

Unfortunately, we lived in an environment where image was everything. I was more impressed with the millionaire who wore earned holes in his jeans than the overnight success who had to prove his worth by wearing expensive fashion. Alan didn't agree. He would have been so much happier with me if I had just looked like the others.

"I'd just like for you to have a normal nine-to-five job and wear corporate suits," he would tell me in a heated moment.

"Not going to happen," I'd inform him. But it hurt. When we'd first met, after I'd gone out on a limb and joined the ski club at college, he'd liked that I was different from the other girls. I had dark brown hair, cut in a shag style, not the straight sun-bleached blonde hair of the tanned California girls. I wore jeans and t-shirts, not halter tops and short shorts. In fact, I found out later that he had first asked about me as "the girl with the sweaty armpits." (Hey, I was nervous!)

I was still dressing pretty much the way I had when he'd first fallen in love with me. In fact, I still had the sweaty armpits (but more from getting older and approaching hot flash territory, not nerves). I hadn't changed much. I didn't really believe that he had either, but at times, I mourned the alternate future we might have had if we hadn't succumbed to the lure of the comfortable suburban life, if we had stuck to our original plan when we were young, idealistic, anti-materialistic.

When we returned from the mall, I stuck the shirt my mom had bought me in the back of my closet, then collapsed on the couch, exhausted. I saw a message on my answering machine from Dr. Williams's office, but I assumed it was a courtesy call to let me know that the lump was fine. It was already late in the day, so I would call back on Monday.

Saturday we returned to yet another voicemail, this one from Dr. Williams himself. What a nice guy. My doctor, my crush, calling me over the weekend to assure me that all is well. I tried calling back, and we began a game of telephone tag. Not to worry. We would talk on Monday.

Early Sunday evening, I came home from a day out on my own. I can't remember exactly what I had been doing. The girls were playing with friends, and my parents were in the family room watching television. They told me that Dr. Williams had called again and would like me to call him at home. I called his home and finally caught him in.

"Hi, Dr. Williams. Are you getting ready for your Jackson Hole trip?"

He was very calm. He had clearly done this many times. "The lump was fine. There was no sign of any cancer."

I sighed and was about to thank him for going out of his way to call me over the weekend, and even have me call him at his home, when he continued. "We did find cancer cells in the milk ducts surrounding the lump."

Pause.

"It's called ductal carcinoma in situ."

Okay. . . .

I guess he thought that would mean something to me. Later I learned that *in situ* is Latin for "in its original place," and *carcinoma*, also Latin, referred to the most common type of cancer, which begins in our tissues. Thanks for that information, Mom, the research queen.

"The lump in question turned out to be fatty tissue," he continued. "But as a precaution, we took some of the tissue from around the lump, and inside the milk ducts we found ten cancerous cells, one less than it would take to officially call it cancer, but enough to call it precancer." We all have precancerous cells in our bodies, and usually they are naturally killed off. But sometimes they multiply and become cancerous.

Silence.

I walked to the front of the house, toward the large wooden staircase off to one side of the spacious entryway. Feeling very heavy, I sat down, hard, on the third step.

"We have options," Dr. Williams went on. "You could wait and do nothing, getting mammograms often, hoping to catch any problems. You could have more ultrasounds and watch the area closely. You could have radiation and monitor the breast after the rounds of radiation. Or you could have another lumpectomy to see if there are more cancer cells in the area."

So, this was intense. I started playing with my hair, concentrating on the wavy brown strands, a habit that usually comforted me.

Suddenly, there was a loud commotion at the front door.

"Hey honey, we're home," came Alan's sing-songy voice as the two of them banged at the door. "Come kiss me. I'm really gross from the mountain. I don't have keys. Let us in."

They were clearly a few beers in and way too happy.

"Let us in!" they yelled in harmony.

I jerked the door open, gave them the nastiest look I could, then walked away to continue talking to Dr. Williams. As I turned away, my arm went out to stop them from coming toward me. I wanted to slam the door in their grinning, filthy faces. Alan and Jon followed me to the stairs.

"Go away," I mouthed to them, glaring. "I have cancer."

Alan tilted his head, his eyebrows furrowed. The left eyebrow with the childhood scar scrunched more than the other, making an oddly curved line. I motioned for them to disappear, and he and Jon tiptoed into the family room. To add insult to injury, apparently Dr. Williams had spoken to my parents earlier in the day and had alluded to the results. His confidentiality breach did not faze me, but I was furious with my parents. Dr. Williams and I decided to continue our discussion on Monday, and I stormed into the family room.

"Why didn't you tell me?"

My father took control, as he always did. "We didn't know everything, so we wanted Dr. Williams to tell you. All we knew was that there was a problem." He was trying to stay calm, trying to diffuse the conversation, but he could tell I was not buying it.

I was angry. Angry at my parents for not preparing me. Angry at Alan for coming home so happy. And angry at my perfect breasts for betraying me.

At that moment I knew my fate. I would go through the motions of doing my due diligence, researching as much as I could. (Let me rephrase that: My mother and I would research as much as we could.) But I knew there was no question of what to do. The choice was a simple one for me. Find out if there was more cancer. Have another lumpectomy. I was not going to take any chances; cancer was inevitable for me, and I had a wonderful life and family that I was not about to lose.

The second time around was not as eventful as the first. All Dr. Williams had to do was unzip the zipper and take out more stuffing. I didn't have to go through the boob wire, which I did not miss.

A second surgery in one month and a future with cancer. I was way too young for this. My fortieth birthday was coming up, and I was determined not to let cancer mar my celebration of the start of a new decade.

Chapter Four

Mountain or Molehill

*D*r. Williams phoned me with the test results. They had not found any more cancer cells. What a relief. The problem now was how to handle the information I had. Yes, there were cancer cells. Yes, they were found in the milk ducts, a common area for breast cancer. Yes, my family history was riddled with breast cancer. But officially, this was precancer, not cancer.

I phoned the National Institutes of Health in DC to see if there were any research programs I could join. My parents had been part of many NIH studies, including those related to my mother's breast cancer and my father's recently diagnosed Parkinson's disease. Unfortunately, the funding for such programs had taken a hit as the economy worsened, and there were no studies to fit my situation. So I was back to my own research, with the help of my mother, the support of friends and family, and many, many second opinions.

"I'm giving you the award for getting the most second

opinions I've ever seen," Dr. Williams informed me. "What have you found?"

"That there is no right answer, no right procedure," I reported.

Our relationship had gone from lighthearted conversations about our outdoor adventures to serious business. My second opinions were all over the map. It was suggested that I do everything from nothing to radiation to a mastectomy. Radiation therapists pushed radiation, and surgeons pushed surgery.

All along, just as with the lumpectomies, I knew what I had to do. I was simply going through the motions to show Alan that it was the right decision for me. With my family history, a family that needed me (and I needed them), and my beautiful breast already scarred, this was a no-brainer.

I would have a full mastectomy with immediate reconstruction, and I would have it as soon as possible. I wanted any sign of cancer out of me, and I wanted it out of me fast. Right then. All they had to do was unzip the zipper that had been unzipped twice already. Easy.

Alan noted that a mastectomy seemed like overkill, but that he would support and love me no matter what I decided. I knew that.

I had to find a plastic surgeon to perform the reconstruction. My HMO allowed me to use any surgeon I wanted, even outside its organization. "It's my fortieth birthday," I would calmly tell each doctor I interviewed. "And I'm having a mastectomy and reconstruction for a birthday present."

Their reactions were as varied as the second opinions. Some were stoic; most were just confused. Some would put their hand on my knee with empathy and just stare. Dr. Jacoby was different right from the start. For one thing, we met in his office, not in an examination room, as with the other doctors.

"What can I do for you?" he asked, just like everyone else. He towered over his carved wooden desk as he gently leaned forward.

As soon as he asked, I started crying. I knew he was the one. He did not take pity on me, but he had the warmth and gentle assurance I needed. I was going to be okay in his and Dr. Williams's hands. I was now in love with two doctors.

During my previous recoveries from surgery, I had grown to love the oversize blouse my mother had given me. It was my comfort shirt, cool, baggy, never needing ironing. The lightweight cotton kept its soft shape without being too stiff.

I was wearing the shirt one afternoon, thinking about the upcoming surgery, when the girls' pet hamster caught my eye. I gently lifted him out of his cage and slipped him into the crested pocket that I had always thought so dumb. The button on the pocket closed just enough to keep the little guy comfortably nestled. He seemed very happy in his little den, traveling around with me. He would move around, fall asleep, wake up, and move around some more.

I began carrying him around regularly, at least for the short time we had him. I would point to the moving pocket and say, "See, I have breast cancer."

I was proud of myself, keeping a sense of humor. I really did have this tangible, alien thing moving in my body, underneath

25

my big shirt. I thought it was funny, but other people did not. The joke was usually met with uncomfortable silence. Alan was speechless at first. Then he suggested that maybe I should see a counselor.

He was doing his best to help me, but humor was how I handled it. I was doing what I needed to do.

Chapter Five

Decorating 101

When we lived in Portland, in my mid-twenties, I worked at Pendleton Woolen Mills, where I met Karren, a fabric designer. She was the West Coast version of Monica Silverman. She had a fantastic lean body and wore cool denim skirts and Frye boots, which I love.

We began having lunch together, and then hanging out socially with our husbands. They celebrated Alan's thirtieth birthday with us, showing up at our tiny apartment in their little red Aston Martin with a six pack of beer.

I wanted to be her when I grew up.

When she told me she was pregnant, I was very happy for her but concerned that this new friendship was fleeting. At the time, I had no desire to be around babies. My career was my focus. But we continued to get together with them, and after Karren gave birth, we showed up at their house, unannounced, right after she got home from the hospital. We'd brought a rubber tree plant. For a newborn.

Somehow, not a baby nor a poisonous plant would stand in the way of our friendship, which only continued to grow. Our families even lived together for a time, while she was going through a tough divorce.

Now, fourteen years later, our friendship was as strong as ever, despite the distance. She'd remarried and had another child, and they were now living in Salt Lake City, her hometown. Throughout the years, our families had gotten together for various outdoor adventures— skiing, hiking, canoeing, white water rafting—in Salt Lake and in Jackson Hole, Wyoming, where they had a condo. During part of those holidays, Karren and I would catch up while Alan took all the kids exploring the wilderness of Wyoming and Utah. When Karren's middle boy was asked, in fourth grade, to write a paper on a famous explorer, he wrote about Alan.

We also spent most of my birthdays together, and this year would be no exception. She was bringing her youngest daughter, four-year-old Aubri. Unlike Karren's older daughter, who was her carbon copy, Aubri's features were larger, a combination of Karren's and her husband's, but she had her mother's light brown hair and clear blue eyes.

As soon as they walked in the front door, Karren insisted on seeing our bedroom. "After your surgery, while you're recovering, when we talk on the phone, I need to picture where you will be." She removed the ever-present pencil from behind her ear, where it had been stationed for the fourteen-hour drive. "We need to decorate your bedroom so I see you in a beautiful place." Aubri followed in step with Karren, fingering her mother's pleated shorts, which had replaced the denim skirts Karren used to wear. She still wore the Frye boots.

I was certainly not opposed to having a beautiful Karren-decorated bedroom.

"I know exactly what you need," she said. "This room is big, and it needs some pattern and color. You've done a great job with the paint color, a typical Lynne 'non-color,'" she laughed, referring to the gray.

This was actually more my style in clothing, not in paint choices. My dining room was coral, and my family room was a deep blue-green, with different patterns of wallpaper. The girls had followed suit. Braiden had chosen red for her bedroom door and green for her room. Her bathroom was red, chartreuse, and peach. She'd also helped pick out the beautiful deep periwinkle blue for the living room. Chelsea had chosen purple for her room, and the playroom was chartreuse and turquoise.

When I'd finished painting the living room, a neighbor had dropped by just to see what color I had chosen.

"Heard you'd done it again," she'd said.

By now I had a reputation to uphold.

Karren continued to examine my bedroom, occasionally pausing to jot down notes. "We can move the bed in front of the fireplace you never use, and the mantle will make the perfect headboard," she said. "There's a great Ralph Lauren sheet pattern with rich jewel-toned colors that we can cut up and sew for curtains, tablecloths, and pillow shams."

It was not in our genes to go out and buy fabric to make curtains. Anything we did had to be created from something it was not.

Karren worked diligently cutting the sheets, matching the patterns, and making the most perfect curtains, tablecloths, and shams anyone could ever imagine. I made the meals and the all-important coffee, which Karren inhaled. Otherwise, I just sat on the floor next to her, talking about everything except the surgery. When we got together, we solved the problems of the world, so during this visit, we solved every problem but mine. It felt good to solve problems other than mine.

Aubri loved hanging out with the "big girls." Even Braiden, usually more of a book-devouring loner, kept Aubri company, along with Chelsea, our social butterfly. At one point, Braiden came in the room, sprawling her tall, unusually thin body on the bed and tapping a steady rhythm on the mattress with her foot. She began braiding her hair absentmindedly.

Soon after, Aubri came squealing into the room, chased by Chelsea, her usual effervescent smile plumping her cheeks. "Aubeeee!" Chelsea cried as she charged. She had a slight lisp, and hadn't been able to pronounce her *r*'s when she was younger. She still dropped them on occasion when she was excited.

The two flounced on the bed, Chelsea's curly red hair falling forward as she tickled Aubri mercilessly. At first Braiden looked annoyed by the interruption, but then her squeaky laughter erupted as she stepped in to gallantly save Aubri from certain tickle doom.

Karren and I rearranged the bedroom furniture a few times to find the ideal setup: "This is where your friends can sit as they talk to you," Karren said once she'd figured it all out. "This is where the kids can play or read while they spend time with you. And this is where you can prop yourself up while watching *Judge Judy*."

She had my life completely worked out in this room. In her mind, my life would exist only in here, the space she had lovingly created.

Chapter Six

Just Another Zipper

With the bedroom decorated, I was ready for surgery. Dr. Jacoby coordinated with Dr. Williams, and all was in place. Again, I arranged for Braiden and Chelsea to go to friends' houses for the first few days, while I was in the hospital, and my parents would come up a week after I got home.

Friends reached out to help in any way they could. Our social circle was young, so I was the first to encounter the dreaded *C* word. We were all setting an example for those who would unfortunately and inevitably follow.

It was up to Dr. Jacoby whether he would do immediate reconstruction or wait, based on how the breast looked after Dr. Williams did his thing. This was my third surgery in one month. It was inconceivable to me that I would have to wait and go through another operation after this one.

Dr. Williams unzipped the zipper and removed all the breast tissue, including the nipple and skin around it. In my research, I had read that the nipple is one of the most common places for cancer to start. If I was going to the trouble of having a mastectomy, I wanted any chance of cancer out of my body. The mastectomy went well, and Dr. Jacoby took over, placing an expander implant into the breast area, under the chest muscle. A tube under my skin went from the implant to under my arm, where it was attached to a small valve that was placed under the skin beneath the armpit. All you could see of the valve was a bump in the skin, about one inch in diameter. This barbaric invention, the expander implant, would be gradually filled with saline, through a needle into the valve, about every ten days to pump up the breast and stretch the skin.

We called this my Arnold Schwarzenegger period.

The surgery went flawlessly, and with the exception of my usual throw-up routine, my recovery was uneventful. I returned home on schedule, and my room was ready for me. All was in place.

I did not feel well, and the pain was terrible, but I assumed this was normal. I had just been through numerous surgeries, and I had not handled any of them without feeling terrible, so I plugged on. This was not going to bother me; it was just a stumbling block. At one point, the pain was so intolerable that I called the doctor, who talked me through removing the extra drain tube by myself. Gross.

My mother called and said that they were, for some unexplained reason, changing their plans and coming up early. They had an evening flight, so Alan planned to pick them up on his way home from work. That day, while the girls were in school and Alan was at work, I picked up a small doorstop. It was not heavy, and I thought nothing of it, but as the day went by, searing pain began to take over.

I was alone and began to panic. As the oddball "creative" in my neighborhood of beautiful housewives, I was not terribly close to anyone—except Brenda, who also did not seem to fit in. Along with our family's rescue dog, Beans, she was my morning walking buddy.

"Hi, could . . . could you come over, . . . now?"

"What's wrong?" she asked, trying to sound calm.

"I don't know, but I hurt so badly."

"I'll be right up. Kelly is here. I'll bring her." Kelly was her teenage daughter.

I unlocked the front door and went back to my bed, where I curled up in pain. I could not breathe. All I could do was cry and try to find a comfortable position. Even the beautiful bedding could not calm me.

Brenda let herself in.

"I don't know what happened," I tried to say, but my voice was hovering on hysteria.

Brenda found a paper lunch bag in the kitchen and had me blow into it to help me calm down and breathe. Slowly, I was able to stop crying. Kelly stood at the end of the bed, frozen, watching this adult thrash in pain.

"I'll call Alan," Brenda said.

Alan got home quickly, slamming the door from the garage into the house and running into the bedroom, piercing dark eyes as wide as could be. He undid his tie and threw it and his blazer on the floor. Beans curled into it, looking for a place to hide.

"What's going on?"

Brenda and Kelly stood to one side as he rushed over to me.

I had gained control and was not panicking. The pain was still terrible, but I kept reminding myself that I had just had surgery, and this was probably normal.

"I don't know," I said, "but it hurts so much. It's swollen and hot, but maybe that's normal after surgery. I feel like such a wuss."

"I can't tell anything either." Alan's face seemed longer and whiter than normal. He glanced at Brenda, puzzled.

"What do you want to do?" he asked. "I don't see anything wrong, and you seem okay now. I don't want to take you to the hospital if you don't need to go." He was not a fan of hospitals and had seen his fill of them in the past few months.

Brenda interjected with her schoolteacher authority. "I think you should take her to the hospital, just to be sure. I'll pick up your parents, in case you don't get home in time."

As we drove, every bump in the road sent excruciating pain through my chest. Alan put his right hand on my leg, driving with his left. He tried to keep his eyes on the road while watching me to make sure I didn't pass out.

The hospital was not yet crowded with Friday night mishaps, and a young intern came to exam me right away.

"What can I do for you?"

"We don't know," Alan began. "She had a mastectomy five days ago, and all of a sudden she's in so much pain, and there seems to be swelling. She did lift something, but it wasn't heavy. We don't know what's going on."

The young intern took a few moments to read the chart.

"Well," he said haughtily, "we really can't tell what's happening here, as you had a plastic surgeon outside of our on-staff surgeons perform the surgery, so how are we supposed to know what is normal for his surgery?"

"I can tell you that I'm in a tremendous amount of pain, and the breast is swollen." I tried to be firm, but the pain was getting in the way.

"How can I tell if it's swollen?" he replied. "*Your* surgeon can't use our emergency room, so he can't come here to see you, so how can we tell? We don't have his notes or know what meds you're on, so what can we do for you?"

I was exhausted, Alan was helpless, and neither of us had any answers for this a-hole.

"Can we call in another surgeon?" Alan suggested. He had always been a great mediator, and he saw that we were getting nowhere.

"Well, I just don't see that it will help, as there is no way to tell if your breast size is normal from the surgery or not. You just had surgery. Of course you're in pain. What do you think happens after surgery?" There was not a trace of empathy in his face. "I can't tell if there is a problem as, I say again, you used an outside surgeon, so I can't see what I can do for you."

Maybe the intern's indignation caused enough frustration to distract me from the pain, but by that point, I just wanted to go home. Alan saw that, and we decided to leave. In hindsight, I wish we had insisted on seeing someone and insisted that they let Dr. Jacoby consult, but I just wanted my bed, a strong dose of painkillers, and my mother.

I climbed into bed, exhausted, in pain, and drugged.

Brenda dropped off my parents, and my mother hurried to my room. She did not notice the beautiful new decor. She probably wouldn't have noticed anyway. She was used to me redoing my rooms, changing everything from paint color to furniture— even the room's usage.

"I knew I needed to be here," she said, stroking my hair. "For some reason, I knew we needed to come now. I just had a sense."

She was not the type to believe in senses in that way, so I was surprised. She could not have been more right. It had been a long time since I'd felt like a little girl who needed her mother. Now I needed to be a child again, comforted by the unconditional love and concern that only parents can give, the reassurance that they will always be there when you need them.

My swollen breast was searing with pain, but the pain-killers began to take the edge off. My room was dark. I felt dark. I had been stoic throughout this experience, and now I was falling apart. I could not hold it together any longer. I wanted my comfy bed to engulf me. I wanted to stay in this beautiful dark room and stop the pain. I felt defeated.

But I couldn't be. I had two young children and a wonderful husband who needed me. *Just push through the pain,* I told myself.

With all of Braiden's health problems, we had established a mantra for when she had to go through something painful:

Close your eyes, grit your teeth, and do it.

It was my turn.

Chapter Seven

Pistachios in the Dark

All that Chelsea remembers of my surgery and recovery was my lying in the dark bedroom eating pistachio nuts. I don't remember the pistachios. What I do remember is neighbor after neighbor coming by, as though I was the pope giving my blessing to the ones not yet touched by cancer. I was moved to know that everyone cared, but they would drop by one after another. It was exhausting.

On one of those days, after watching some TV, then reading a bit, I found it hard to get my eyes to focus, so I was starting to doze off when I felt a presence in the room.

I hazily opened one eye.

"Oh, you're awake." It was one of the skating moms. Braiden's regular ice-skating had gotten both of us involved in the skating world. It was a land of unrealistic Olympic dreams and crazy stage moms. Her long limbs, bird bones, and tiny features made her the epitome of a classic ballerina when she was ice-skating, which by now was almost every day, but she did it for the love of skating. She was practically oblivious to the cutthroat competition.

I wished I could have remained oblivious to the woman standing at the end of my bed, holding a plant.

"Uh, I guess I am," I mumbled.

"I brought you this azalea plant," she said, holding it out in front of her. "Well, we got together and bought you this plant. Tina, Sherry, Rachel, and I. We were so concerned about you. It was my idea." She finally realized I wasn't going to sit up and take the plant from her and set it on the dresser. "Kathi wanted to let you know that she would have bought this for you, but she wasn't asked, so it's just from Tina, Sherry, Rachel, and I. Just in case Kathi says anything to you about who bought you the plant. She was pretty mad that she wasn't included, but it's just from us."

Always drama at the skating rink.

Another time I was dozing off when I looked up to see a neighbor I did not know very well staring down at me. She was also holding an azalea plant. What was it with the azaleas?

I received many phone calls, including several from a local cancer support group. A representative wanted to come over to tell me about all the wonderful services her organization provided. I asked her not to come, because I had all the support I needed, but she would not listen.

"Honey," she said, "I know you have friends and family who love and support you, but our organization provides help that we would love to share with you."

Okay lady, calling me honey is not going to help you here.

It was the same conversation every time she called, and she

called often. My mother and I continued to assure her that we were fine. The woman would not have it.

One day, she showed up on my doorstep, unannounced. If she had truly understood what I was going through, she would not have done this. How could she come unannounced and unwanted? In a moment of weakness, my mother let her in.

She had brought a basket of flowers, information on support groups, brochures on the latest mastectomy-related products, and a much-too-happy grin on her face. I had grown to hate much-too-happy people.

"Here we have a lovely brochure about the latest sleeping bra," she chirped. "It's really helpful for the large-breasted woman."

Yes, I'm wearing a baggy T-shirt, but please, lady, how can you not see that I am far from large chested? At least give me products I can use!

I was having a hard time with nausea, so I was up and down, rushing to the bathroom constantly. I thought this would be enough to dissuade her from staying, but not a chance. Every time, I returned to her relentless enthusiasm and concern. My mother and I finally convinced her that she had done her job and could leave.

Big Brother of the cancer world must have sent a message to everyone about my surgery. I continued to receive calls from support groups, as well as various cancer organizations and institutes. Fred Hutchinson Cancer Research Center called to ask if I would participate in a cancer research study. Being the child of the Olympians of medical research participation, I agreed.

Two women came to my house with a list of questions. I had to answer the questions quickly and was not feeling well. I wanted them gone.

"When you were eight, what was your diet?"

Really? Was this really what they wanted me to remember right now? I could not tell you what I ate an hour ago, let alone what I ate as an eight-year-old.

"I liked butter. Cooked peas with butter." That sounded really good to me right then.

They wrote it down.

"My mother had cancer, and many aunts and cousins have had cancer," I volunteered.

They did not write that down.

The remaining questions were pretty much the same. This was for the birds. I was surprised, because Fred Hutchinson is known to be one of the best research centers, and these questions were ridiculous. Honestly, do you remember what you ate as a child? I mean, I remember various foods, but do I remember enough to make it a valid representation of what I ate? Probably not.

I received a summary of their conclusions, which were basically that I had cancer because I had eaten too much fat as an eight-year-old. Not that nearly every female member of my extended family has had breast cancer. No. *I ate too much fat as an eight-year-old.* I will admit that my diet might have been a factor, but it certainly was not the cause! My faith in medical studies was seriously wounded.

Soon my notoriety in the neighborhood wore off, and everyone went back their lives. But then a neighbor I was not particularly close to brought over a chicken casserole that changed my life. It was sheer ambrosia. In my baggy pajamas, I would stand in front of the sink, looking across the backyard at the distant Olympic Mountain's never-melting glaciers, glimmering in the sunshine. With the largest spoon available, I would inhale pure edible comfort straight out of the cold casserole dish. The comforting smooth texture of the creamy sauce combined with the spectacular view enveloped me in a bubble of calmness in what had become an uncertain world. Later I asked for the recipe, and to this day, the casserole is our family's comfort food.

If I learned anything from this experience, it was that kindness means the most well after a traumatic event. One of the best things you can do for people going through a crisis is to think of them after the commotion has died down. That is when they need you to remember them.

Chapter Eight

Waking My Inner Dolly Parton

The recovery seemed to take forever. I could not understand why I was having so much trouble getting back to normal life. Every ten days, I would go to Dr. Jacoby's office, and he would inject more saline solution into the valve under my arm. The injection did not hurt, but as the skin was stretched to create a breast, the pain returned. *Of course it hurts,* I told myself. Skin that had only recently been cut open was being tormented.

After each injection, I would spend the next few days in bed on painkillers. It did not make sense to me that I could not handle the pain. After all, I had given birth to two children without any drugs at all; I was woman! Nonetheless, for eight months I went through this routine: saline injection, three days in bed, constant pain for a week. I developed what I called my 4 P.M. headaches. Every day, at 4 P.M. Pacific, rain or shine, summer or winter, I got an excruciating headache. Of course, this coincided with carpool time, but I was not about to let anything get in the way of carpool. That was my chance to see my girls interact with their friends, to have fun with them and eavesdrop on their lives. I learned so much about them during that time.

I became depressed. I had battled depression before and briefly taken antidepressants, but now I was trying to stay off them. I was too tough for that. I could manage it myself. And what in the world did I have to be depressed about? Other women had gone through this. I could not understand why I was having such a hard time. Painkillers helped, but as much as I wanted to become an addict, I had a reaction to every painkiller I took for more than three consecutive days. I tried going without painkillers, rotating painkillers, but nothing seemed to help.

After eight months of hell, my breast looked fantastic. I had been pumped up to twice the size of the other breast. The pumped-up breast would remain that size for some time to stretch the skin. During this time, I became an expert at adding rolled-up pantyhose and shoulder pads to one side or the other so my chest would look balanced. Eventually, my doctor would remove some of the saline so that the skin and breast would have the "proper droop" of a normal breast. After all, everyone needs proper droop.

After pumping it up and letting it down, they would remove the valve, create a nipple by folding some skin into a nipple shape, tattoo the area around the nipple, and voilà—I'm beautiful. I told Dr. Jacoby that when he tattooed my nipple, the least he could do was tattoo a rose or something cool. He disappointed me when he said that he would not do it. He explained that he wasn't a tattoo artist.

So before my next visit, I drew a lightning bolt and cloud on my breast with felt-tip markers. When he came into the examination room, I threw open my blouse to reveal my masterpiece. I had lost every bit of modesty with this man. He had already seen more of me than I could have ever imagined.

"Wow, if I had known you were an artist, I would have thought about doing this for you."

He was impressed. I was disappointed. I would have loved a pretty souvenir of my troubles.

My breasts looked great. Except for the large zipper across the top of my left breast, you could not tell the fake from the natural one. It had been a tough road, but the payoff was worth it. Except for the depression, constant lethargy, and 4 P.M. headaches, I was back to normal.

From the time Braiden was a baby, it had been clear that I needed to stay home with her. She was always home with some health problem or off to the doctor or ER. On top of her severe allergies, she was injury prone as well, constantly spraining her ankles. I doubt any of her elementary school teachers can remember a day she was without her crutches. She was grace in motion on skis or skates, but once she got her feet on the ground, she was an accident waiting to happen. We even rigged up a pulley system to get her crutches easily from the main floor to the top floor and back again. She decorated the ropes with ribbons and lace.

So while she was still quite young, I had quit my full-time clothing design career to work from home part time, developing small lines of clothing that I sold to such stores as Nordstrom (a Seattle-based company most locals knew as Nordies), as well as to small boutiques and by word of mouth.

"It seems like your designs coincide with whatever phase the girls are in," Alan once joked. "Before they were born, you designed baby announcements. When they were born, you designed baby clothes, then outerwear for toddlers."

He was right. Although for years, Braiden had worn nothing but dresses (white dresses, no less) and mismatched shoes and socks, the girls and I were now wearing lots of sweatshirts, so I decided to make a line of silk-screened shirts combined with crazy leggings (which were popular at the time). I created colorful illustrations to print on the sweatshirts and even went so far as to sew some of the garments myself. I hated sewing, but this was a cost-efficient way to go. I mixed and layered vibrant patterns on top of patterns. The outfits sold well, for girls and for women. I would wear the shirts, but I never had the nerve to wear the leggings. I was still most comfortable in jeans and sweats.

I was the neighborhood Bohemian, still the "eccentric" one in the neighborhood, but it had been about eighteen months since my mastectomy, and new families had moved in, so Brenda and I began organizing a party for everyone to get to know each other. I was also the carpool queen and loving every minute of it. On some days, I would put 150 miles on the car while working on my ventures, or taking Braiden, Chelsea, and friends to their classes and activities. I kept an open bag of coffee in the car because the aroma helped keep me going. I don't drink the stuff, but I love the smell, the look, and the consistency. I love making coffee, and I even love the sound it makes when hitting the bottom of the cup, but I hate the taste.

Around this time, Chelsea surprised us all by announcing she was going to try out for the basketball select team.

"Okay," I said, confused. She had never shown any interest in playing basketball beyond the casual, fun level. The kids trying out for this team had already been singled out as talented. They were already on teams together, with coaches who took the sport seriously.

Alan no doubt had flashbacks of coaching Chelsea's basketball team when she was younger. She had just loved running with the ball. It didn't matter which way she ran. She ran up the court and back, a huge grin on her face, not caring which way was defense or offense. Just running and dribbling was good enough for her.

"Shoot the ball!" the parents of our team and I would yell.

"Stop the ball!" we'd yell as she ran down the other end of the court.

But it was never in our family's nature to tell her not to try. So try out she did. We weren't allowed to watch, but I drove her to the tryouts and waited outside. There they were, the skating moms of the basketball world. Discussions consisted of how many basketball camps the girls were going to this summer or what offense or defense had worked in the last game. There were definitely leaders of the pack, and the mothers clearly knew where each girl ranked on the basketball pyramid. No way was Chelsea going to break into this world. These kids had started their career long before Chelsea had figured out that this was a competition, not just a fun game.

But if there's one lesson I have learned about Chelsea, it is to never underestimate her. She made the team, and I was so proud of her, but I couldn't help but groan inwardly at what I was in for with my new group of moms.

In this way, our everyday suburban lives went on, but beneath the surface, I still felt terrible. My 4 P.M. headaches would not go away, and I felt a dull pain and depression all the time. Some days I would get everyone off in the morning and head back to bed, sleeping as late as 1 P.M. I also had abdominal pain and worked with my family doctor to relieve that and the depression.

"Last year, all the meds I was taking began with a *P*," I observed at one visit.

My doctor cocked his head a bit, as if to say, hmm, had not noticed.

"Well, I guess this will be my *C* year," I quipped.

He looked at the list of medications we had decided I would try. "Guess you're right. I hope the *C* year helps."

Chapter Nine

Inside Out

My father's health was declining. My younger sister, Lauren, had moved in with them to help, but the effects of the Parkinson's were becoming more and more apparent. Through his connections from the many research studies that he and my mother had participated in while living in DC, he was able to get into a study that involved injecting stem cells into the brain to see if they would reproduce and help the brain regenerate. The study was based out of Columbia University in NYC, but NIH in DC was monitoring the study, and the actual operation would be performed in Denver.

I flew to Denver on my own. The operation took much longer than expected. It was very painful, but my father tried to keep his sense of humor. We didn't know who got the real stem cells and who got a placebo. We would not know until my father's death, when they would perform an autopsy on his brain. But deep down, we all just knew he would get the stem cells.

Lauren had stayed in San Diego, where she was also helping our parents build their dream home on the beach. Jamie came up from Colorado Springs, where she lived on a ranch with her husband and son, along with Jamie's menagerie of horses, dogs, llamas, cats, turtles, and any other animals she could get her hands on. We had an odd family reunion, eating family dinner in the hospital cafeteria and sharing memories while standing over my father, who had one of those metal halos around his head to keep it still. The hospital stay was short, only two days, so we all quickly returned to our lives, hoping that this would be the answer to this terrible disease.

I continued to struggle with the pain and depression, so acting as my own shrink, I decided it might be good therapy to take a sculpting class. I did not have any sculpting abilities, although as a child I had carved turtles out of bars of soap. I have never been good at attending classes either. I got kicked out of Girls Scouts because I never went to meetings; as a college student, I skipped lots of classes; and as an adult, I hadn't done any better, but I was hopeful that I would follow through with this class.

The studio was on the second floor of a two-story storefront in an older area of town. It felt artsy and quaint. The class was small, so the instructor could spend quality time with each student. We were allowed to work on any clay project we wanted, and most students wanted to learn how to use the potter's wheel. That was not for me. I wanted to sculpt.

With my sweatshirt illustrations, my style was cutesy. I hated that no matter how hard I tried, my artwork ended up cute. So I was surprised when I sculpted a human head that turned out to be anything but cute. It had a glazed look of despair, gazing into nowhere. Now, where in the world had that come from? The instructor had helped with the technique, but the head had created itself, with me just following its lead.

"That's a haunting figure head," the instructor remarked.

She was right. I had not paid much attention to it as I was creating it. I had just let it happen.

"Does it have any significant meaning to you, as to why you made it so haunting?"

I pressed my lips together and thought about that for a few seconds, trying to conjure up a story of love lost or something. "No," I finally replied. "It's just what it is."

I did not like it, but it drew me in. It was not worth finishing it other than to fire it.

"I'd love to buy it from you," she continued.

I was shocked that she thought it had any value, but I needed to keep it. I realized that it represented my private pain. I could not share that with anyone.

It came home with me and hid behind other knickknacks. Every once in a while, it would peer out from the corner, but I would never really look at it. Just a glance before moving along. He (don't know why he was a he) haunted me. I hated him. I was not a collector of stuff and would think nothing of passing something along to someone who would get pleasure or use out of it. It was surprising that he stayed.

My breasts were beautiful, so I was feeling complete on the outside, yet lousy inside. But I had come to terms with this dichotomy and lived with it, even starting to get out of my comfort zone with the clothes I wore. I had a job interview for a part-time freelance position as a clothing designer, and I decided to use a personal shopper at Nordstrom. I did not usually shop there, but Nordies seemed like the most likely place to find clothes that would say, "I'm a professional yet artsy woman—take me on!"

Nordstrom was in an exclusive mall in Bellevue, the "nouveau riche" area of Seattle. The mall had started long ago with Sears and JCPenney, and remnants of these origins were still there despite attempts to create a snobby, upscale image. Nordstrom was a special world. The familiar piano player was always there, playing happy tunes to stimulate our shopping experience. The smell of coffee wafted from the stylish coffee stand.

The personal shopper's office was in the corner behind the Givenchy and Chanel evening gowns. I was intimidated yet at home. Although I was not part of the couture fashion world, I knew it and understood that these were just clothes that a laborer had painstakingly created for minimum wage or less.

"Is there a special event you'd like an outfit for?" the shopper asked. She was somewhere in her late thirties or early forties, and she seemed nonjudgmental. I was comfortable with her.

"I have a job interview as a clothing designer, and I need a professional but creative outfit," I explained. She must have thought it odd that a clothing designer would need help with her own clothing, but I had designed menswear, children's wear, and outerwear, and at least I had the sense to know that most of my designs would look terrible on me.

"Let's get you going, and we'll knock their socks off," she said confidently.

I was open to whatever she suggested and ended up spending far more than I had ever spent on clothes before. As I describe this outfit, please remember that it was the early nineties. She put together a plaid blazer, with shades of deep violet, yellow ochre, and black. Sounds hideous, but it was a subtle plaid, and the fit was perfect. She paired that with a black pencil skirt, black tee, black tights, and low black suede heels. I was hot!

A few days later, I met the owner of the clothing company at a downtown private men's club. He was impressed and flew me to his offices in San Francisco, where I met the other designer. It was a perfect opportunity. Only one problem. When I arrived at the offices, the designer was confused about why I was there. Turns out the owner had forgotten to tell her that he was thinking about adding another designer. She put the kibosh on that idea real fast. That was the end of that, but now I had a new look, and I was ready to go on to the next design opportunity that presented itself.

Then one morning, I woke up to find my new breast swollen. It felt like it was the size of a watermelon.

I phoned Dr. Jacoby's office. "I look like Dolly Parton on my left side." My voice was calm, but inside I was a nervous wreck. I started playing with my hair. Gray was rearing its ugly head amid the dark brown, and the gray strands felt kinkier than the others.

The nurse, who knew of my headaches, pain, and depression, went to talk to Dr. Jacoby, then came back on the line. "Can you come in ASAP?"

Chapter Ten

Farewell to Thee, Dolly Parton

*L*et's see what we can do with antibiotics and bed rest, but I'm worried." Dr Jacoby looked at the nurse then back at me. "If the swelling doesn't go down in five days, we will have to remove the implant."

That was not going to happen. I had worked too hard, and it looked too good. Unfortunately, my breast did not agree, and five days later, in Dr. Jacoby's office operating room, my breast and I would part ways.

Brenda drove me to and from Dr. Jacoby's outpatient clinic because I had not been able to get a hold of Alan. The doctor gave me a mild sedative, and I was awake the entire time. He removed the implant with no trouble, and luckily, it had not leaked. I started to feel pain and discomfort as he scraped the remaining breast tissue away from my chest. I could feel the pressure of the scalpel and hear the scraping, like fingernails across a chalkboard. I felt sick and defeated.

He was taking away what I had endured so much to keep.

My instructions were to go home and rest. There was nothing more to do.

As a footnote, after my mastectomy, the FDA had come out with a warning regarding the type of implant I had. It was apparently so problematic that it was then taken off the market.

As we drove home, my body was, as usual, not happy with the anesthesia.

"I need a Pepsi," I insisted to Brenda. "Could we please stop and get a Pepsi?" I thought it would help settle my stomach.

It didn't. Sorry, Brenda.

"Pull over, quick" became a repeated request, every few minutes. The three-mile drive home turned into a marathon. I stopped to throw up every few minutes, and in between stops, I cried.

"I'm not going to be able to help you with the party tonight."

"Well, duh," she replied, trying to bring some levity to the situation. As if she needed to. It was no doubt a ridiculous scene to anyone following behind. This brand new monster of an SUV stopping and starting on small residential roads as what appeared to be a soccer mom repeatedly leaned out of the car to throw up.

Brenda helped me crawl into bed, and when Alan got home, I really cried. My perfectly reconstructed breast was gone. I had been defeated, which I never took well. I was stubborn and compulsive, yet my fight to keep my breast had come to an end. Losing a breast was hardly the worst thing that could ever happen,

I tried to tell myself. Until this moment, I had not allowed myself self-pity, but now I was feeling pretty sorry for myself.

I insisted that Alan, Braiden, and Chelsea attend the neighborhood party.

I wanted to be alone.

Chapter Eleven

Life Lopsided

The 4 P.M. headaches were not as constant. I had more energy. It was gradual, but I was feeling better. Physiologically better, anyway, but lopsided.

The HMO ordered a prosthesis for me. It did not matter to them if I had a breast or not, or that I had made such a valiant effort to keep the breast they had paid for. It was all routine for them.

They referred me to a specialty store in Bellevue, near the Nordstrom, but not in the mall. The store was in an area that was still being transformed into its new upscale image. Twenty-story glass-walled office buildings and condominiums were rising into the sky with such rapidity that every day, a new obstruction seemed to appear along the horizon.

The makeover had forgotten this store. Tucked between the uber-contemporary multiuse buildings, amid the cranes creating the new face of Bellevue, sat this one-story, one-store building, painted off-white with blue trim. It had its own parking lot, something not available anymore in most places. It might have been someone's house long ago, with its cedar roof and double Dutch doors. A small sign hung above the doors. You could easily miss it, which I guess was the point—to be discreet about such subjects as missing boobs in this town of the beautiful people. I thought I might find comradery in commiserating over missing body parts, but no, the building and I were just two isolated objects out of place.

Close your eyes, grit your teeth, and do it.

With a deep breath, I opened the small white double Dutch door to my new life.

I had walked straight into the fifties and was greeted by another relic of the same era.

"Hello, how are you?" She was old. All the employees were old. They wore too much makeup, as if they were hoping the layers of foundation would cover the years of wrinkles, but the makeup only made the winkles more prominent. The hairstyles were frozen in time and in place—coiffed, set, and sprayed to death, never to move again. Their hair looked freshly dyed in my favorite red/brown noncolor, but I did catch glimpses of gray, indicating it was time for a beauty parlor appointment. I wish the hair dye companies would come up with a better "old lady" color. Maybe purple.

Their outfits were just that—outfits, ensembles. Not a casually chosen blouse and a skirt, but put-together, purposeful outfits, which did not mean their choices were great. Polyester suits, with polyester ruffled blouses peaking from the jacket. The colors of their clothes were artificial, just like the breast prostheses they sold—baby blue, a pink that should not exist.

The entire building and its contents were artificial.

"My HMO sent me here to get fitted for a breast prosthesis," I said calmly, trying to keep any emotion from showing.

"Well, dear, you are in the right place."

Here we go again with the honeys, sweeties, and dears.

With a look of pity, she gestured for me to go into the dressing room and undress. She would return to help me. The other saleswomen were rigid and cold, looking away from me as if I did not exist. Their commission was gone. I was of no use to them.

I had not been this uncomfortable in . . . ever. I was about to undress and expose my lopsided, scar-ridden chest. The skin where the implant had been was saggy now that it had no breast to conform to. Ripples of skin lay across my chest, joined by a fatty mass that extended from under my arm, where the bulb for the pumping-up sessions had been.

I undressed and waited. I had not worn a bra because my remaining breast was small enough to get away without one, and of course I had my baggiest clothes on. I was in my overalls phase and looked like a hillbilly, which did nothing to impress the sales staff. I was one of those pathetic underclasslings contractually sent to them by the bourgeois HMO.

It seemed an eternity.

"You're a B cup. Right?" She took out a measuring tape and wrapped it around my chest. The tape fell ungracefully into the area of the missing breast. "We can fit you into a B cup, or we can increase the cup size and provide you with an insert for the other side so you can be larger . . . and look so much better."

She was checking out my chest while trying to assess and re-create me. Never had I been more exposed.

"No, thank you," I responded timidly as I covered my chest. "I think I'll stay a B cup."

"Whatever you say." Her obvious disapproval showing, she turned quickly to get the prosthesis.

"Here you go." She unceremoniously handed me a heavy pink twelve-by-twelve-inch box with a photo of a woman's face on it, straight out of the fifties—blue eyes, classic red lipstick, and perfectly styled blonde hair. Her head was tilted slightly, with one manicured hand delicately cupping her chin. She was blissfully at peace. Written in a soft white that blended gently with the soft pink of the box was "A Woman's Happy Experience." A hinge at one end of the box opened to expose the neatly packed silicone breast lying on top of a plastic form, which cupped its treasure perfectly. The cardboard was much heavier than that of most boxes today. They had spent a lot of money on that box.

Who where they kidding? This was a cold, plastic excuse for a woman's missing body part.

I gently lifted the prosthesis from its nest and was surprised by how heavy it was.

"It's anatomically correct in every way," the lady proudly pointed out.

It was sort of an almond shape and had defined sides to it. The side that went around toward the underarm was elongated to mimic the muscle that wraps around the chest. The top tapered out to give a nice line toward the décolleté area, and the bottom had Dr. Jacoby's precious proper droop.

"It's heavy," I smirked, trying to interject a bit of lightness into this stodgy old lady.

"These are made to be perfectly correct in every way, even to the correct weight of your breast," she haughtily explained.

Oh joy. The least they could have done was make the stupid thing lighter so we could weigh less than we did when we had breasts.

The prosthesis comes with triangular pieces of Velcro, about the same size as your breast area. First, you remove the protective paper from the sticky side and smash it against your chest, positioning it where you hope the breast will look most natural. Then, you take the breast out of its very special box and smash the Velcroed side of that against the Velcro fabric attached to your chest. Instant breast.

But the weight of the prosthesis pulls the skin away from your body, even with a size B, so a bra, which I hate wearing, is mandatory. And even then, since the breasts are not well attached to your body, your bra is not quite anchored under the breast, so slight migration ensues. Nothing is in place, but nothing is out of place, and everything is uncomfortable.

Supposedly, the triangular fabric can stay on your body for up to five days, even when showering and sleeping. But if you try this, it feels like a constricting super-sized Band-Aid across your chest, pulling at you as you move. And if you wear it in the shower, it feels like a wet clam and starts to unstick, even if you had just put it on that day.

I tried to wear the prosthesis without the Velcro, but I was always scared that this synthetic creature would pop out of my bra or get a mind of its own and move to a place where it felt more comfortable. This was my future. The prosthesis was expensive and uncomfortable, but I told myself that in time, I would learn to love my new buddy.

The level of discomfort for what I got out of it made no sense to me. Summers were especially hard, as my chest sweated beneath the unbreathing bag of silicone. I wore the prosthesis as little as possible and turned to my baggy clothes to hide my lopsidedness.

What surprised me most was how much I hated being lopsided. It had been two years since the start of this crazy journey. On one side was the well-worn zipper, which had been opened three times with nothing to show for it, just saggy skin and a fading tattoo. I dreaded taking showers; I hated looking at my lopsided body. I hated washing my chest and toweling off, and I especially hated looking in the mirror. It was a constant reminder of what I had fought so hard to keep and had lost anyway.

I was getting regular mammograms for my other breast, where the doctors were constantly finding suspicious lumps. The fear of cancer was a constant. I had had enough. I went to my beloved Dr. Williams, and we decided it was time to take the other breast. With my history and new lumps, it made sense. It had been six months since losing my implant and two years since the original diagnosis—a drastic move, yes, but we all agreed it was the right thing to do.

With my history of having surgeries to celebrate holidays, I used this as my Valentine's Day present. Oh boy, a new zipper! I was hoping he would put this one below my breast.

Here I was again, lying in the operating room, waiting to

be put to sleep, questioning what in the world I was doing, by choice, no less. Knowing my usual reaction to surgery, I wondered if this was the dumbest move I had ever made. What would happen if something went wrong and I died? My children were young; they needed their mom. This was really stupid. I was more scared than I had ever been. And, to top it off, for the first time, I was missing my children's events.

This was not necessary. Yet I knew it was.

"How're you doing, honey?" the nurse asked as she gently touched my thigh.

We had seen each other so often that I guess we were finally close enough to use those endearing names.

The doctors and I knew the routine. The surgery went well. It was over; I had no more breast to give. With my history, Dr. Jacoby would not consider the possibility of using implants. He was right. I was devastated.

I was about to be very flat.

Chapter Twelve

The Rise of Annie Flats

Back to the prosthesis store and my favorite ladies. I decided to stay with my natural cup size, A/B.

"Very well," Miss Prissy muttered. "Your choice."

I could hear them thinking, *why in the world would she do that?* This was my opportunity to be any size I wanted. Why would I not want to be as big as possible? But I liked being small. My breast size was the only small thing about me. With little fanfare, I received two pink cardboard boxes, two anatomically correct and accurately weighted breasts, and two bags of Velcro Band-Aids.

I continued to wear overalls, sweatshirts, and baggy tees, and I began to question whether you could tell I had breasts at all. The prostheses spent more time in their boxes. Alan did not seem to mind, and I told myself I was saving money by not having to buy the expensive Velcro strips.

In an organic progression, I stopped having breasts. I felt liberated. I did not have to wear a bra! Unless they are very large chested, most women take off their bras as soon as they get home. I did not even have to put one on! Being flat became a personal statement; I could still be a woman even if I did not have breasts. Gloria Steinman would have been proud. This was my fashion statement. I had the control to define myself as a woman, just as I had control to change my name.

The Good.

I began taking dance classes. I would throw a baggy tee over a leotard, and off I would go. I could jump, run, twist—do anything I wanted—and not have breasts flopping around like the other women in the class. I stayed cooler too.

The Bad.

I was self-conscious about hugs. Do people expect to feel a bra when putting their arms around a woman? I wondered if they were surprised not to feel one. Did people wonder where the breasts were when they hugged me?

And the Ugly.

My chest is gross. The skin that used to be a breast is now a rippled mess of saggy scar tissue and skin, definitely an improper droop. Sometimes it seems like there is so much drooping that it makes a breast. Believe me, it is not. In addition, the faded tattooed nipple is still there, but way too low. On the other side, where I had the latest mastectomy, the skin is fairly flat and smooth, almost concave. Dr. Williams was considerate enough to put the scar on the bottom of my chest. Thank you, Dr. Williams.

I started experimenting with the color of my now-graying hair. It started out innocently enough, but I think Braiden and Chelsea eventually started a betting pool: "What color will Mom's hair be today?"

"Mom, you need a dye job" was Chelsea's friendly reminder to keep the pool active.

I went from dark brown, my natural color, to streaks of blonde, to more blonde, and on to the ever-so-popular and memorable red phase. Not a natural red, as I had wanted, but a bright pinky red.

One week, the gray was slowly overtaking whatever color I had in, so I decided to go platinum. Short, spiky platinum hair with huge overalls.

Nice image, soccer mom.

Life returned to our "normal"—a revolving door of activities and people. I purchased a Suburban truck. (I know, I know, we were *not* going to be one of those suburban, materialistic, gas-guzzling families, but the purchase would be justified later.) We could fit lots and lots of kids into it, so I returned to being carpool mom, complete with my open bag of coffee.

Fall was soccer season for Chelsea, one of the many sports involving balls that she loved. Although Braiden was an avid ice-skater, Chelsea had the more rugged athletic body, and the personality to match. As a child, she'd never walked—she always ran, hopped, or skipped from place to place.

We went to all the games, many of them early in the morning. Seattle is not the driest place on earth, so the soccer fields were often covered in a dense fog, which usually burned off around halftime. The moms came up with creative outfits to deal with the cold, wet weather.

"Love the neon one-piece suit you found," a mom would comment.

"Where did you find the deep-sea fishing suit? I simply must have one," another would squeal.

We layered the outerwear over long underwear and polar fleece. As the fog dissipated, we would shed each layer until, by the end of the game, we were left wearing clothing that was actually appropriate for being in public. For me, the more layers the better. My overalls and sweats were perfect.

In keeping with Alan's observation regarding my clothing lines, a walking friend, Mary, and I decided to start a line of promotional garments for sporting events. We would customize sweatshirts, T-shirts, and other items with an event's logo and then sell the items at the event. I would create unusual logos, which would distinguish us from the many other companies similar to us. We bought a machine to press the design onto the garment, purchased massive amounts of sweats, tees, and hats (on top of my own never-ending supply of baggy clothes), packed them into my Suburban (see, this is why I needed the Suburban), and off we went. But we still had not agreed on a name for the company.

It was during one of our walks that the perfect name hit me.

"I know this name is crazy," I blurted, then turned timid. "But what do you think of Annie Flats? It's a wide spot in the road in central northwestern Washington State, named after Alan's grandmother. She was the postmistress on the Indian reservation where Alan grew up and was a huge part of his life. It's just a funny name. You can be Annie, and I can be Flats. After all, I *am* flat."

We looked at my chest, the ground, and each other.

"I love it!"

The sun peaked out from the morning fog. Annie Flats was born. Our company grew quickly. I handled the creative and manufacturing end, and Mary handled the business end. As I was the public face of the company, people assumed that my name was Annie Flats, and lo and behold, Annie and Ms. Flats were added to my repertoire of names. Really. They thought my last name was Flats. I liked the name Annie, so I went with it. It stuck around for a long time, but eventually, I returned to boring Lynne. It was just too much work and confusion to be two different people.

Soon it became clear that our friendship was more important than our partnership, so we decided that I would buy her out and venture forward on my own.

In this new partnership, I was Annie, and my chest was Flats.

Chapter Thirteen

Strength in Numbers

Over the next few years, we amassed a collection of cars: the Suburban, an SUV that was getting up in miles, an old Camry, and a convertible VW named Ollie. It was a car menagerie. We saw our local mechanics so much, I affectionately referred to them as "my guys." The environmentally conscious hippies of the Pacific Northwest we had once imagined ourselves to be had succumbed. Here we were, with four cars (one of them enormous), living in a huge house in the land of Microsoft multimillionaires.

We also had a menagerie of pets, from our dog Beans to Braiden's grumpy cat, Suki. We had an unintentional habit of naming our pets after food. Maybe it was a tribute to Braiden's food allergies.

Braiden's health stayed fairly under control thanks in part to the cold air of the ice-skating rink. I loved the rink partly because I could bundle up in clothes. I tried to stay away from the skating moms as best I could. One exception was Gail, who had moved from Los Angeles with her daughter, a talented skater who had been paired with a boy from Seattle. It was common for a girl to move to where her partner lived. There were many more girls than boys, so the boy usually dictated the location—just one more part of the skating world that I wanted my daughter to avoid. Although Gail and her daughter were in Seattle for only six months, we became close friends. They would end up moving to Sun Valley, Idaho, and then Kentucky, but in the years to come, I would visit her often, and her Sun Valley home would become my special place.

Braiden's skating coach brought skaters from all over the globe to train in Seattle. The visiting skaters needed places to stay, so we offered to house them and ended up with yet another menagerie—of people. Alan described our house as a revolving door and me as the Kool-Aid mom. I figured it would be fun to get to know skaters from around the world, and it would be good for Braiden and Chelsea to learn about different cultures. Who knows, but maybe this is where Chelsea obtained the wanderlust that would one day take her all over the globe.

Our entourage of skaters came from England, Japan, Canada, Australia, and various places in the States. At one point, six skaters from Australia and their parents came. Between my girls, their friends from school, and the skaters, we literally had people sleeping in our hallways. Hotel Hanson was in full force, and I was in heaven. I would drive the entire lot of kids to skating, basketball, soccer, music lessons, and school. I made large batches of pancakes and waffles for breakfast, and baked ziti became a staple for dinner. Alan taught the kids how to fly-fish.

Trent, one of the skaters from Australia, was obsessed with all our gardening equipment. Because we had a full acre of manicured lawn, we had a riding lawn mower, which Trent loved to take apart and put back together. We also had a branch chipper, which Trent called our "chippa."

"I'm headed out to work on the chippa," he would cheerfully announce.

"Have fun and be careful," I'd yell as he headed outdoors.

"No worries," was always his answer. Loved that: No worries.

I was thrilled because the yard work was mainly my job, and I hated it. Trent adopted us as his U.S. family, called me Mum, and returned many times to stay with us as he trained. His mother visited often as well, and we instantly bonded. They became a part of our family.

Another skater, Ty, would also become family. He started training at the rink when he was twelve, and at fourteen, he went through a growth spurt, surpassing even Braiden in height. Around that time, he also began staying with us. It worked well because he was around the same age as Braiden and Chelsea, so they were able to attend the same schools.

Thin and graceful, Ty moved like a dancer even when doing the most ordinary things. On one of his first mornings with us, Alan came into the kitchen to find the counter transformed into a ballet bar, where Ty was dutifully doing his stretches. Alan was not exactly in touch with his feminine side, so this was a bit uncomfortable for him at first, but as time went on, Ty and Alan became very close, and stretching at the kitchen ballet bar became a morning ritual for the two of them.

Ty's mother was also dealing with breast cancer, so Ty and I bonded over cancer and ice-skating. His mother was not as lucky as I was. He was sixteen when she passed away.

Chapter Fourteen

Mona Soup and Matzo Ball Soup

In the fall of 1997, when Braiden was a sophomore in high school, she began to sleep more and more and was not able to keep any food inside her. The phone calls from school became more and more frequent.

"I need to come home. I don't feel well."

I figured she was like many skaters her age, becoming anorexic and depressed. I was not going to let my daughter fall into the trap so many young girls did, harming themselves to live up to our society's values. I had bucked those values regarding breasts, and I was determined to help my daughter do the same regarding her own body image.

It came as a shock when the psychologist and our family doctor informed me that she was fighting some sort of physical infection. Unfortunately, every test came back negative, and Braiden got sicker and sicker. During her junior year, her five-foot-seven frame was down to ninety-eight pounds, and she attended school only twenty-nine days. She was prone to dark undereye circles due to her allergies, but now her almond eyes seemed sunken into them. Her skin, ordinarily the color and texture of a pearl, was chalky, accentuating the circles even more.

We were all at our wit's end.

We knew that something serious was happening, and we were handling it in our own ways. Alan's way was denial. Chelsea tried to escape into school and her activities. I rearranged furniture.

When Alan got in late, he would trip over furniture in the dark that had not been in that spot when he'd left earlier that day. He learned quickly to turn on the lights in a room before entering.

I closed my business to stay home with her. I was not sorry to give it up. It was a no-brainer. She needed me, and I needed to be there.

But I kept the name Annie and a supply of baggy sweats and tees. Braiden and I would pile on the layers, hiding in the folds of the baggy clothes. Maybe if I layered enough, my deformed body and my worry for my daughter would disappear.

I became an expert at making matzo ball soup: Jewish penicillin. If we ate enough of it, I reasoned, all would be well.

At one point, I thought a kitten might bring some laughter into our home, so on the way back from one of Braiden's many doctor's visits, we stopped to see what was supposed to be a blue point Siamese kitten. I had always wanted one, and Braiden was thrilled at the prospect of having a kitten to curl up with.

We had battled rush hour to get to the breeder's house, and Braiden was exhausted. She didn't even have the energy to fidget with the car radio. She always fidgeted with the radio.

The breeder greeted us in a long dress, which hid any indication that there was a figure underneath it. Her house was filled with plastic flower wreaths, with Enya playing in the background. We followed her into the living room, where three kittens were playing.

"Here they are." She motioned for us to sit on the floor if we wanted to see them.

Two were red point Siamese, and one, who seemed to stay off in a corner, was a beautiful striped grayish brown, but definitely not a blue point.

"I was under the impression that you had a blue point," I said calmly, but I wasn't happy. Braiden looked ready to collapse.

"She is a blue point," the lady insisted.

I don't know what drugs this lady was on, but judging from the bongs around the room, I could guess.

I wasn't going to argue with her, so I picked up the tiny kitten. *No wonder this lady can't see what color she is,* I thought. The poor kitten had almost no hair. Her belly was distended, and her right clubbed foot was bent from the ankle joint inward. She had six toes on three of her feet, including on the club foot.

The kitten was a sorry sight. To make matters worse, the lady proudly pointed out the old-fashioned pop-bead necklaces on the kittens to get them used to wearing collars, but she had obviously forgotten to add beads as the kitten grew. The necklace was way too tight around the pathetic kitten's neck. Braiden and I looked at each other in amazement. This lady was supposed to be a reputable, responsible breeder. She was anything but.

"That one is $150," the breeder proudly stated. "Isn't she cute?"

She was endearing, for sure. This tiny, pathetic, club-footed, hairless creature wasn't what we'd come to see, but she needed us, and we needed her.

"I can't pay that for a kitten with a club foot" was my starting point. I was trying not to say, "This kitten is a mess, you irresponsible woman; just let me rescue her."

"I'll take $80."

"She will need to go to the vet, and I don't know how much she'll need. We'd give her a great home."

I don't think the offer of a great home did any good, but the thought of vet bills probably did. She finally agreed to give her to us. Braiden ripped off the pop beads as we left.

We named her Mona Soup, which was a name Braiden had made up when one of her friends was making a film and asked what her stage name would be. To this day, there is a film out there with Mona Soup in the credits.

The next day I took Mona Soup to the vet. "It was very nice of you to take the cat in," she said softly. "But her club foot is inoperable, and she'll live only a few weeks. At least you'll have her and she'll have you for that time," she said softly.

I was devastated. I was losing my daughter, and now our family had to watch this poor kitten die. It was unacceptable. I would take her home, and we would love her and make her well.

Within two weeks, little Mona Soup was growing hair, and the distended belly was giving way to a healthy, full belly. Her clubbed foot straightened out within just a few weeks. It was a sign. She was going to be okay, and so was Braiden. I just had to keep going, keep making matzo ball soup.

Chapter Fifteen

Multiple Personalities

With my business gone, I was going stir crazy. *Learn to paint,* a little voice in my pea brain said. I had never considered myself a fine artist, but for some reason, this made perfect sense.

I would teach myself to paint the hardest subject—children—in oils. If I could do that, I would consider myself a painter. I needed to be home all the time and did not want to take classes. My parents had always taught us to just go out and do it, so that is what I did. I read every book and magazine on painting that I could get my hands on. I worked every minute and enjoyed every second. I was prolific, but now I needed homes for all these children I had painted.

An article about a young girl with an incurable disease caught my attention. Friends of the girl's family were organizing an auction to cover her medical expenses. I offered a painting for the auction. Then I found other organizations to donate my work to. It took me out of my own worries and myopic world. People who attended the fundraisers started calling to see if they could buy one of my paintings. Never one to turn down the opportunity to make money, I launched a new career. I started attending art fairs and got my work into a few small galleries.

My art and my ongoing quest to figure out what was wrong with Braiden were my jobs. And my passions. I was part-time Lynne, part-time Annie, part-time nurse, and part-time artist. Some of the time, I would use Annie as my name, and sometimes I would be Lynne. Some of the time I would dress with my flat chest proudly displayed, and sometimes I would hide in the baggiest outfit I could find. No one, not even me, knew who I was.

After a year of watching Braiden deteriorate, we found a doctor who could help us. She had two major infections in her intestines, and somehow everyone had missed it. It took another year of pins and needles, but with the help of a creative school curriculum, she was able to graduate with her friends and go off to the college of her choice in Maine.

With Braiden away and Chelsea and Ty busy with their lives, I was able to devote all my time to painting, and the paintings continued to sell.

"Have you painted today?" Alan's small fingers would wrap around the door opening, as though he were feeling if it was safe to come into the room. He could tell when I hadn't. I was, as he put it, "impossibly grumpy."

Too true.

We spent hours in our family room, which had been transformed from a meticulously decorated gathering space to a multifunctional room, with me painting away at my super-sized easel while Alan sat at his brand new fly-tying desk, concentrating on the latest technique.

"Your paintings are beautiful, but it's time to push yourself and find your own style," he commented one evening.

"I know. I've been feeling that way for a while, but I'm surprised you noticed. I didn't think you paid attention."

I put my new olive green wing tip glasses on.

Alan put on his coke-bottle-thick frameless glasses.

We went back to our obsessions.

My opportunity came when, for my fiftieth birthday, I was given a condo in Sun Valley for one month. With my Suburban fully loaded, I set off with Beans and my bike for a month of self-exploration. I was spending less time as Annie and more time as Lynne. My paintings got more abstract, and more colorful. I switched my subject matter to horses and women in evening gowns. Funny how all the women were flat chested.

The house emptied out. Braiden was still in Maine, Chelsea went off to college in Connecticut, and Ty moved to New York City to skate with the prestigious Ice Theatre of New York.

Life was continuing on.

Chapter Sixteen

The 9/11 Snowball

*Y*ou wouldn't think the tragedy of 9/11 would affect Seattle, but it hit hard. Just one of Seattle's employers laid off over thirty thousand people. The ripple effect hit us, and Alan too was laid off. We had two girls in private colleges, a large mortgage, me with minimal income potential, and Alan, middle-aged in corporate America—too experienced for some jobs, and too old for others.

"Maybe it's time for a drastic change." I was pacing across the family room, wrapping and unwrapping a strand of my now very gray hair around my finger. Alan listened as his gaze followed the graceful line of his fly-fishing pole. With his head bent down, I could see the spreading bald cap that had started out years ago as a barely noticeable bald spot at the crown of his head.

"If we're going to be unemployed somewhere," I continued, "it might as well be in a place that we love. We've always hoped that someday we would move back to a ski town." In 1973, as newlyweds, we'd lived briefly in Telluride, but the oil embargo and a terrible drought had made it impossible to make a living there. We'd always planned on returning to that shared dream, to living the simple life of ski bums in a small town, but we'd ended up taking the not-so-simple path up the West Coast to raise a family in the Pacific Northwest.

I stopped pacing and stood in front of him until he looked up from his fishing pole. "Maybe," I said. "This is our time."

Alan's eyes teared up.

We narrowed our choices down to Ashland, Oregon, or Bozeman, Montana. Bozeman had been our first choice as newlyweds, twenty-seven years ago, but we had not been able to find jobs there. Maybe now was our time. Alan's cousin Les lived in Bozeman, so with his help, we visited a few times to scope out job and housing prospects.

Then we put the house on the market.

"You need to paint your living room beige," the Realtor dictated. "The periwinkle will be a deterrent in selling the house."

My house was not beige and never would be beige. By now I had accepted who I was. My life, my body, and even my house would never conform, not even to sell the house during this terrible time.

We sold our house in one day, to a wonderful Iranian family. The extended family came to look at the house together, and when the grandfather, a little man, gingerly stepped into the living room, he looked around, sighed, and with a soft smile said, "Blue. It's blue."

You would think that this would have been a tough time, but for me, it was liberating. I donated and sold almost every piece of furniture we had, and we went from a full house to thirteen pieces of furniture, including beds.

"How are you doing, dear?" the neighbors would pathetically ask. I was ready to get out of there, *dear*.

With a smile from ear to ear, I would respond, "Great! I'm having the time of my life getting rid of all this stuff. We've sold all but two of our cars" (yes, I sold the Suburban), "we've furnished a home for a nonprofit organization, and we've either sold or given away just about everything we own. It feels great."

I meant it.

Luckily, Braiden and Chelsea were back at school, so they did not have to see their past flying out the front door. I felt sad about leaving the house that I loved and had raised my family in, but I was ready for a new adventure.

It was one of the most liberating times for me in my healing process. The ugly clay head I had sculpted after my first mastectomy appeared from where it had been hiding. It was time to purge whatever this ugly head stood for. I took it to the backyard and smashed it into the rocks. Surprisingly fragile, it shattered into tiny pieces.

I walked away, not feeling a thing.

We negotiated to stay in the house through the end of the year so that we could have one last family holiday there. Braiden and Chelsea came home to say good-bye to their friends, the house, and Seattle.

We had to be out of the house by January 5. On December 24 we had not yet decided where to live.

On December 26, I announced, "We're moving to Bozeman. It makes the most sense. We know it better than

Ashland and love it. Are you guys okay with that?"

It was a statement and a question that I did not want an honest answer to. Of course they did not want to move. This was their home.

"We're with you guys." Braiden and Chelsea did not even look to see if the other agreed. "We support anything you decide to do."

I love my children.

Chapter Seventeen

Moving On

*J*anuary 4.

Alan and I put Chelsea on a plane for a semester in Prague. Braiden and her friends would continue to load the U-Haul. All of our family possessions fit into a seventeen-foot-long truck.

That night, Braiden, Alan, and I slept in our empty 4,500 square-foot home on a couple of mattresses we were giving to friends. We were lost in our own thoughts. I hoped that Braiden was thinking about her upcoming semester in Paris rather than leaving her Seattle past behind.

January 5.

Alan, Braiden, and I took off for the 750-mile drive to Bozeman with our dog, two cats, two cars, and the U-Haul truck. Alan drove the U-Haul in the lead; Braiden followed him in the old SUV; and I brought up the rear in our Camry.

Bozeman had been in our lives for over thirty years. In fact, Alan's parents' family was originally from Montana, even though his mother's tribe, the Okanogan, was based in north-central Washington State.

At a rest stop, I kidded Alan, "You're coming full circle, going upstream to where you began. You're just like a salmon."

Oh, if I had only known then what I was saying.

January 7.

We then drove 750 miles *back* to Seattle in time for Braiden to run in the Olympic Torch Relay and then board her flight to Paris.

January 8.

Finally, we drove 750 miles back to Bozeman to start our new life.

Whew!

I had strategically rented an apartment that we would not want to stay in. Yes, I said *not*. Located on a small triangle of land between the highway, airport, and train tracks, it was noisy and would motivate us to purchase a home as quickly as possible.

I found a job right away as an administrative assistant in the International Programs Department at Montana State University. My art career would have to be placed on hold. I had given up any notion of being Annie, or anyone else but Lynne, yet the feeling of empowerment I'd felt exploring who Lynne was artistically when I'd gone to Sun Valley was quickly fading into resignation. Now I was "just Lynne." The job, which called to mind all the international ice skaters who had stayed with us in Seattle, seemed promising. I was working in an office now, so my wardrobe had to change from baggy sweats to baggy dresses.

I was comfortable with that.

It would only be a matter of time before Alan found a job, so we started looking for a home to buy. It had always been my dream to live in a city's funky downtown area, and now was the time. I found my spot in what Bozeman called the historic district, an eclectic neighborhood with mansions and shacks on the same street. We closed escrow on a wonderful Craftsman home the day before Chelsea was to return from Prague, right after Memorial Day. Braiden would come home a day later.

We were planning on building an addition to the attic, so we left the bulk of our belongings in a rented storage unit since the house would be in turmoil for a while. Our new home was furnished with one sofa, a table, a television and stand, and two beds. To complete the ensemble, we found a lovely side chair with burgundy-and-beige stripes at a garage sale, and Alan purchased an exquisite overstuffed chair and ottoman for me as an anniversary present. It was huge, soft, and squishy and could easily sit two adults, or one person could curl up to read or drift off to sleep, enveloped in downy comfort. A fanciful all-over pattern of coral poppy flowers with olive leaves softly coordinated with the off-white background. It was pure serenity wrapped up in a chair. We placed it in our sunroom. I painted the walls a deep coral, which accentuated the bright white trim and built-in bookshelves that were above the windows on all three sides. It was our bright, sunny getaway.

The house had one story and a basement, which had a two-bedroom apartment we could rent out to college students. The attic was huge, and we planned to add bedrooms and a bath upstairs. The rent would pay for the remodel, but for now, we would wait until Braiden and Chelsea went back to school. We wanted to enjoy the summer with them.

After the girls arrived, we spent one pleasant evening in the backyard, surrounded by beautiful trees and chirping birds. The smell of the salmon cooking on the BBQ wafted with the breeze. Children played soccer in the park behind us.

"This place isn't bad." Chelsea was applying sun block to her face. Her squishy nose and ears were already turning red.

"Let's go to Yellowstone tomorrow," Braiden suggested. It was only an hour from Bozeman—right in our backyard, in Montana speak.

They seemed okay.

I sighed. We had done it.

I settled into my potato sack dresses and sweats and put my flat chest out of my mind as the summer quickly turned to fall. With the girls back in school, we rented the basement to three graduate students from India. We often spent delightful dinners together, deep in conversation, comparing our cultures and foods.

We began remodeling the house in late October. The plan was to create a staircase at the end of the living room and push out three dormers into the roof to create an entirely new floor. We had made new friends through the local synagogue, where we also met our builder, Paul, a soft-spoken six-foot-four man who had moved to Bozeman years ago instead of going to law school. Alan and I were to act as general contractors and do as much as we could ourselves to save money, while Paul guided us through the process.

The first thing we had to do was remove mounds of insulation from the attic. Alan and I donned white one-piece "zoot suits" and full-face masks, and then, using buckets, we began removing the insulation.

"You look like aliens," Jay from downstairs commented.

Alan gave him a small smile and planted a kiss on my slightly exposed lips. He had not been this happy in thirty years.

Around this time, Alan started a job as VP of manufacturing for a small company. He would go fly-fishing during lunch, after work—any chance he got. My job, however, was taking its toll. I was feeling more and more stifled. I was as comfortable with my body as I could be, but inside, I was restless.

"This job is killing you inside," Alan commented one day after work. "Your spark is gone."

Maybe it was time to return to my life as an artist.

Chapter Eighteen

5:30 p.m., Friday, January 17, 2003

*B*raiden and Chelsea spent the winter holidays with us before Chelsea, our wanderer, flew off to Kenya for her spring semester. It was a lot cheaper for her to fly out of Salt Lake City, so Braiden, who had another two weeks off from school, and I took this opportunity to drive her there and visit Karren.

Alan could not take the time off work, so he said his good-byes to Chelsea from home. He was used to saying "good-bye for now" to her. He would meet her in the spring to climb Mount Kilimanjaro for her twenty-first birthday.

"Love you. See you in May." He kissed her good-bye and gave her a huge hug, and I noticed that he was now only a few inches taller than she was. He was getting shorter—and a bit pudgy, which was showing up in his face as well, making his eyes look even narrower, although no less piercing.

He turned to me now for a quick hug good-bye. Even with a few extra pounds, he was still in great shape, still strong. He'd easily shed the weight during that season's mountain climbing and skiing, I figured.

"Drive carefully," he said. "I'll see you Friday around dinner."

We had tickets for a film festival Friday and Saturday nights.

"No problem," I said. "I'll see you then. Love you."

They looked so cute, the three of them. I took a photo of Alan with his girls, and I could see his eyes twinkling underneath the tears. He was so proud yet so sad to see Chelsea go.

"Love you too." Then he hugged Braiden, told her he loved her, and we were on our way.

It was a six-hour drive to Salt Lake, but there was snow and ice on the road, so we drove carefully. We enjoyed our staple driving music: Rusted Root, Dirty Dancing, Havana Nights, Ricky Martin—only dancing music on road trips. I think the car bounced as much sideways as forward from our wiggling bodies.

"You have your passport, inoculation papers, phone numbers, ticket, malaria meds, asthma meds, and extra prescription?" I rattled off the list we had gone through so many times that she rolled her eyes as she nodded. I was nervous about her going to Kenya with her asthma, but I was not about to tell her she could not go. She could handle herself.

We spent the night with Karren, and then we all went to the airport early the next morning to send Chelsea on her way. Her overstuffed backpack barely made it through the baggage check, but she flashed her famous smile to the check-in attendant, coyly playing with her curly locks, and somehow the backpack made it.

"How would you like to drive up to Sun Valley and spend the weekend with Gail?" I asked Braiden as we were heading back out to the car. It was a three-day weekend for me, so there was no rush to get home.

"Great idea! But what about your film tickets?"

"I'll call Dad. He could invite Les or his friend Larry to go."

As I expected, Alan did not mind at all. He knew that I loved Sun Valley and had not seen Gail in a long time. It was hardly out of the way, only an extra six hours, which was nothing. Braiden and I would be home Sunday afternoon.

Gail's daughter had moved to their extended family's home state of Kentucky, so it was just the three of us. Three silly, giggling girls having a pajama party, except for one brief moment, at 5:30 P.M. Friday, when I felt a quick knot in my stomach that said, "Do not go home yet."

The entire drive home on Sunday, I stewed about my job and decided it was time for me to get back to my artwork full time. I was sure that Alan would support me; he saw what I needed.

"Are you excited to get back to school?" I asked Braiden as we drove through the desolate high-altitude desert of eastern Idaho. We could see the magnificent Grand Tetons off in the distance. The mountains were more ragged than most of the Rockies, and both Alan and I had a special love for them, as we had skied, and he had climbed, those mountains many times.

"I really miss Keegan," referring to her boyfriend at the time. The two of them where on the phone constantly. "I can't believe I'm about to graduate. Everyone keeps asking me what I'm going to do, and I haven't a clue."

"That's okay," I responded while writing the script in my mind of how I was going to present my idea to quit my job.

By now Braiden's constant wiggling was about to drive me crazy. It was either her feet or her hands. Constantly. I had yet to hear a full song on the radio the entire trip. I finally turned it off when I saw her hand reaching for the tuner buttons for the millionth time.

We arrived home, and an overexcited Beans greeted us. Les was on the sofa, which was no surprise. He was often there. But I did not want him there today because we were tired and I had important stuff to talk to Alan about. We said a polite hello to him, and I looked around for Alan.

"Beans, get *down!*"

Les stood up and walked over to us.

"Alan is gone," he said, voice cracking. Les was a big man with a bellowing voice. This was not his voice.

"Gone? What do you mean gone?" I was totally confused and getting more and more annoyed with Beans.

Braiden started to panic. She began waving her arms, wrists flapping about, hopping in place. I reached my arms around her entire torso while looking at Les, still not understanding what he was talking about.

"He's g-gone. He had a heart attack last night." He tried to keep his voice calm and collected, but as our conversation went on, he started to lose control.

"Dad! Dad. . . . Dad, where are you." Braiden pushed my arms away and started jumping around in circles. I grabbed her and held her as tightly as I could. Her silky long hair melted around her face as her head collapsed onto my shoulder. She sobbed uncontrollably.

"What do you mean?" My grip was getting tighter and tighter. "Beans, get *DOWN!*"

"Alan asked Larry to go to the movies with him last night," Les explained. "Larry showed up at 7:30 and no one answered. The house was unlocked, so he went in and called to Alan, but he didn't answer, so Larry went home. But he kept calling Alan."

Les's voice quivered as he looked toward the floor, planting his feet firmly to steady his giant torso. "He called this morning, and still no one answered, so he called me. We came over to the house and we went in. . . . We found him in the shower. He was gone."

Les gave a whimper and turned away from us to sit down on the garage sale chair. The chair groaned as Les's massive body slumped into the cushions.

I held Braiden as tightly as I could. Arms twisted around each other's bodies. I was still totally confused.

"We couldn't find you," Les said. "No one knew where you were, and we had no phone numbers. I called everyone you know in Bozeman, and no one knew where you were."

"We were in Sun Valley," I responded shakily. "I called and told him where we were going, but he was the only one who knew."

My thoughts went to Chelsea, on her way to Kenya. How in the world was I going to get a hold of her? I needed to get to Chelsea. *Now.* I needed to hold Braiden. I needed to understand what had just happened.

"Braiden, do you remember where I put Chelsea's contact

information? I know I have her contact information somewhere. Where is it? Where is it? *Where is it?*"

My boss, Norm, knew everyone in the International Study
Programs. Maybe he could help me find her. He answered the
phone as if he were waiting for my call.

"Norm, can you help me find Chelsea? She is on her way
to Kenya. The program is through St. Lawrence University in
New York. I have the phone number somewhere, but I can't
find it. Norm. Is he really, really, is he really?"

I started sobbing uncontrollably.

He already knew what had happened. Everyone in
Bozeman knew. Everyone but us.

"I'm so sorry, but yes, it's real," he choked.

Les took the phone and made arrangements to get Chelsea's number. By now it was late at night, but Norm was able to
call the program director on the East Coast and get the phone
number of the school in Kenya. I called the headmistress there.
Chelsea had just arrived and was sleeping. We agreed on a plan
for her to call Chelsea into the office in the morning, and I
would call and tell her the news.

It was inconceivable to me that this was how my daughter
was to hear that her father had died.

*What do I do next? This isn't real. I have no experience
with what to do next. Next. I don't know what to do next. Hold
Braiden. Next.* I just saw empty in next.

I made a few of the dreaded phone calls, first to Jamie,
Karren, and Gail.

I asked Jamie to call our parents. It would be too much to
tell them.

5:30 p.m., Friday, January 17, 2003

Jamie and Karren would arrive on Monday. My mother and Lauren would come a few days later. My father's Parkinson's had advanced to the point where he needed to be in an assisted living home and, with his failing health, he would not understand what had happened, so it was best to let him stay home. Gail would be up in a few days. We phoned Ty, who went into "I'm not going to deal with the reality of this, but what can I do to help?" mode and phoned more family and friends.

Then Braiden and I sat on the sofa in the empty living room, waiting to call Chelsea. The hours through the night were still. I tried to take in everything that was happening, but I still could not comprehend what was going on. Braiden understood. Braiden always understood. Through her life-threatening allergies and illnesses, she had a clear understanding of life and death.

I held her as tightly as I could. Every blanket in the house was wrapped around us. We did not say a word. We just watched meaningless TV shows. I could feel her grief through her body. My feelings revolved around confusion and worry for my daughters. How in the world was I going to tell my daughter that her father was gone? Over the phone, no less.

We had to make the call at 3 A.M. to catch Chelsea at the coordinated time. I held Braiden as I spoke. I heard Chelsea's voice collapse. I felt Braiden's body collapse. I knew our hearts had collapsed. I held Braiden tighter and tighter, as she wrapped her long arms and legs unceremoniously around me. It was all I could do. I wanted so badly to hold Chelsea, but I could not. I could not do anything for her but get her back to me as soon as possible. She was alone. I was helpless.

The headmistress had already booked a flight home, and Chelsea was on her way to Bozeman a few hours later. It had taken her three days to get to Kenya, and it would take her two and a half days to get back. It tore my heart apart to think of her on the plane, all alone. Chelsea's college in Connecticut helped with the plans to get her back to the U.S., which meant that all her college friends knew of Alan's death. One of her friends, who was home in Wisconsin, drove three hours in the dead of winter to the Minneapolis airport to sit with Chelsea on her layover.

She finally arrived home. I will never forget her face. Jet lag from flying to and from Kenya for six days, along with three days of crying, had made her face so swollen I could hardly recognize her. But I was relieved to have her in my arms. All I wanted to do was hold on to my children.

Chapter Nineteen

Care Bears and Casserole

It did not take long for the house to fill up. Karren and Jamie were already here and were talking in a corner, Jamie with her back to me but her head turning as she scanned the room, her solid body tensed, clearly ready to take charge if necessary as more and more people arrived. She had very intense brown eyes that seemed to look right through you, but when her gaze fell on me, they softened with such pain that I almost didn't realize I was looking at myself in her eyes.

Four of Braiden's friends from Seattle had piled into an old Toyota Corolla to make the twelve-hour drive, and Braiden's boyfriend and his sister had arrived soon after. Then Chelsea's friend from Seattle came, and my mother and Lauren arrived. The house was a sea of mattresses, with narrow aisles in between. We brought our poppy chair into the living room, where Karren curled up in it. Everyone had fallen asleep, including Braiden and Chelsea, both in my arms. I held on tight, entwined on the oversized sofa, and stared at Karren, snoring away. I wished I could sleep like that. I wished

I would wake up and that this would all have been a dream.

The entire town of Bozeman, especially members of the synagogue, was there for me. It was such a strange feeling for everyone to have known before I did. So many people commented that they had seen Alan that day, at the local co-op grocery store, outdoors, all around town.

"We were out walking and ran into Alan as he was shoveling the sidewalk," a neighbor commented. "We stopped and chatted. Everything seemed great. He did mention that his shoulder was a bit sore, but after shoveling snow, whose isn't?" No one thought anything of it, not even him.

It bothered me so much that I was the last to know.

At least I didn't have to worry about feeding everyone. Friends brought over food, tons of food: salads, enchiladas, casseroles and more casseroles. Braiden, Chelsea, and I put together some of Alan's favorite clothes and bought Care Bear stuffed animals to be cremated with him. The kids had always had Care Bears growing up. By sending them with him, they were making sure he would have us with him. Chelsea picked out her favorite Sunshine Bear, and Braiden her favorite Grumpy Bear. When she was younger, she would transfer all her pain to Grumpy Bear. I picked out Love-a-Lot Bear. Jamie took them, along with some of his favorite clothes, to the funeral home. His parents, who had arrived earlier; Braiden; and I went to see him to say our good-byes. Chelsea chose not to see him as she had said good-bye before leaving for Kenya. Probably a smart idea. He looked so good, which made it even harder to understand.

The days that followed were a blur, with everyone gradually

returning to their lives. After two weeks, Braiden and Chelsea each decided to go back to school. They were certain it was what their dad would have wanted. At the end of the semester, Chelsea would climb Mount Kenya and spread some of his ashes there. He would like that.

The calls to friends became a familiar routine.

"Anyone but him," they would exclaim with confusion. "He was the epitome of health. A mountain climber, skier, backpacker. He was always so active. He was the last person anyone would think would die of a heart attack."

It was hard to hear and so true. Anyone but him.

I went back to work—probably not one of my best decisions. My house was an empty space, under construction, and I thought it would be good for me to get out every day. It was not. I found myself in a pattern. Mondays I was able to make it through a full day at work, but as each weekday went on, I was leaving earlier and earlier. By Fridays, I was only able to make it until noon. I cried constantly at the office but found the house to be my sanctuary.

Fortunately, other university employees donated vacation time to me, and I was able to take the time off without loss of pay. I was not making much, but every little bit helped. Bozeman and its population were taking care of me. The town of Bozeman was like that neighbor who had brought the chicken casserole three weeks after my mastectomy. They remembered me.

Paul, our builder, took over the general contracting work until I could think a little more clearly. When I took it back over from him and started calling contractors, they would ask,

"Are you the lady whose husband just died of a heart attack?"

"Yes, yes, that's me."

"Don't worry. We'll take care of you."

At first I was afraid that taking care of me meant taking all my money, but I quickly learned that they really wanted to help me in my very tough position. That's Bozeman!

One day, I came home from work to find a sign outside the mudroom entrance saying not to use that door. Paul came out looking distressed.

"The floor of the mudroom collapsed," he muttered nervously. "I was walking through it, and it just collapsed. It's completely rotted."

Even though he was standing two steps above me, his six-foot frame looked small.

I peered around him and looked at the large hole in the mudroom floor, then looked back at him, dazed. "Okay," I said. "So what do we do?" All I wanted to do was put on my baggiest clothes and go to bed.

"Um, I didn't expect you to be so calm, but this is good. I've already called the restoration company, and they'll be here tomorrow."

"Okay. I'm going to bed now." I retreated into my sanctuary.

Little did he know how well the drugs were working.

It was January. In Montana. Paul helped me put tarps over the three huge holes in the roof that were slated to become dormer windows. It was snowing hard, and the tarps kept blowing off, but they helped a bit. The mudroom was getting fixed.

For the first time in my life, I had no appetite. My friends helped me muddle through each day to get from point A to point B. The renters downstairs took turns checking on me, and when they saw that I was having a tough time, they sat with me. For where I was, I could not have been in a better place.

My job was going steadily downhill. I loved the university and the people in the office, but I was going deeper and deeper into depression. One day, as I was walking across campus in a blinding snowstorm, it hit me. Never in a million years did I think I would be a *widow* living in isolated *Montana*.

This was not supposed to happen. Alan was the epitome of a healthy lifestyle, a mountain climber and skier who worked out almost every day and ate healthily.

This was not supposed to happen!

I lay in bed, pondering the situation as the tarps flapped loudly on the roof. Here I was, relatively new to Bozeman, in the middle of winter, a widow with two girls in private colleges, a mortgage, a low-paying job I was unhappy in, three holes in my roof, no life insurance, and did I mention no husband?

And did I mention that I had no boobs? No longer was I secure knowing that I had a husband who loved me no matter what my body looked like. I was a widow now. What if—

No, I would not even go there. But, what if . . . I were to date?

What the hell do I do now?

Chapter Twenty

Just Close Your Eyes, Grit Your Teeth, and Do It

I knew I had to do something.

I quit my job to make it as an artist. I figured I could always flip burgers at McDonald's if need be. After all, it would not pay much less than what I had been earning at the university.

In addition, I came up with this great plan.

"What if Dad comes up here to live?" I had checked out assisted living homes in Bozeman, and they seemed wonderful—at a third of the prices in California. "It's perfect, Mom. He needs me, and I need him. And you can come up here as often as you'd like because we will be saving so much money."

My mother and Lauren agreed that it was a plausible idea, and after Lauren grilled the home as to the level of care he would need, we made it happen.

I quit my job in May. My father moved to Bozeman. Braiden graduated and decided to spend time in Bozeman while figuring out what to do. Chelsea got a summer internship with a local international nonprofit organization. Ty moved to Bozeman as an ice-skating coach. We would all be together.

We were all catching our breath.

"When do I have to check out of this resort?," my father would ask as he traded off using his walker and riding in his wheelchair while the girls and I took turns pushing him.

"No, Papa," one of us would explain. "This is your home. You can stay here as long as you'd like."

"Good. I like this."

My mother spent weeks with us and hours with my father, now able to just enjoy his company without being drained by the overwhelming burden of his day-to-day care. Braiden and Chelsea helped out with him, and we all took turns spending quality time with him and with each other. It was the perfect solution for everyone.

We decided my father needed a cat to keep him company, so we found a wonderful older cat whose owner, another resident at the home, had died.

"I like that," he said when we mentioned the idea. "I'll name him Nincompoop."

But my father could never remember the cat's name, so we changed it to Pom, which was short for Pomegranate because he was as fat as a pomegranate.

Then after only three weeks, the facilities manager called one morning. "Your father needs to leave our facility immediately," she said.

"What happened?" I asked in a daze. She had woken me from an unusually deep sleep. "We moved him into your facility because you assured us that he could stay there no matter what his health was and as long as he wanted. I don't understand."

"The cat is causing problems."

I felt terrible. My father loved the cat, but he needed to stay in this facility, so I would find a new home for the cat.

"That's not good enough," the administrator told me. "Your father needs to leave too. We can't take care of him anymore. He needs to leave immediately."

They were a private company, so they could do anything they wanted. I would worry about the fight with them later. Right now. I had to take care of my father.

I was able to find a great home for Pom, but finding one for my father was not so easy. The choices in Bozeman were limited, but we wanted to keep him here. He was happy, and my mother was flourishing back in San Diego.

The only place that would take him was a nursing home. He wasn't ready for that, but the only other choice was to bring him into my house, which was too dangerous with all its stairs and quirks. We had no choice. The nursing home wasn't pretty, but the care ended up being outstanding; the staff was working there because they wanted to, not because it was the only job they could find, as had been the case in San Diego.

His moving day was sad. Braiden, Chelsea, and I tried to put the best light on it, but my father was confused about why he was leaving his resort. But he was a very social man, so he was soon immersed in the small town life of Bozeman, where he became something of a celebrity in town. Everyone knew my father.

We walked with him downtown, and he attended local parades as well as high school and university sporting events. The local ski area had a wonderful program that enabled disabled people to ski, and he was by far the oldest person participating. Other skiers considered it an honor to ski with him.

He was out there every week. "Hey, Sid, great day for skiing!" fellow skiers would call from the chairlifts. People would yell and wave to him, and he would beam. Some would stop to sit and chat with him on the outdoor deck, where he enjoyed his usual after-skiing meal of chili and French fries.

In the meantime, I was managing to make a living as an artist. I showed in local galleries and traveled across the country attending art shows. I put thirteen thousand miles on the car in one summer, traveling from Bozeman to California, to Oregon, and to Kentucky, where Gail had moved to be closer to her daughter. The art shows were exhausting, but I was good at them. Braiden, Chelsea, and Ty came with me when they could; otherwise I was on my own. Setup and tear-down was a challenge.

This brought my persistent clothing problem back to the fore. In Montana, the summers were relatively short. As I traveled to hotter climates, I became increasingly self-conscious. I wanted to look nice, but the less I wore, the more I was of aware of my breasts, or lack thereof; yet the more I covered up, the more hot and sweaty I became.

In addition to needing new clothes, I needed a new car. I no longer had my Suburban, and our old SUV had over 250,000 miles on it. So I took a large canvas with me to the car dealerships and bought the smallest SUV the canvas would fit into. This was car number three. I could not bear the thought of selling our old SUV, as it was a connection to our past. The Camry was too small for art shows, and I kept it for the kids. We were unintentionally back to having a car menagerie, complete with another set of "my guys" to handle repairs.

Home was filling up again. I had three twenty-something kids living with me, I was able to work at what I loved, and almost everyone was healthy. Unfortunately, Beans, our dog, was not faring well. He was a rescue dog that had been abused, and he was now fourteen and in pain. With much sorrow, we had to put him down. Shortly after, Suki, Braiden's cat, had to be put down. With each part of our past vanishing, the pain of losing Alan would be revisited.

But Mona Soup carried on.

Chapter Twenty-One

Where in the World Is Chelsea Hanson?

I was feeling good. My art was going well, and the kids were in good places. It was winter, so the nagging clothing problem was out of season, my body hidden under sweats. My lack of boobs was a nonissue. Comfort was the name of the game.

Chelsea graduated and continued to do what Chelsea does, exploring the world, popping in and out of Bozeman. Her latest was a three-month journey throughout Southeast Asia and India.

Her first stop was Bangkok, where she would meet up with the sister of a friend from Seattle. From Bangkok, they were scheduled to go to Phuket.

I awoke to the phone ringing.

"Hi, Mom. It's Chelsea."

"Hi, honey." It never occurred to me to be worried. It was around 3 A.M., and I was foggy.

"I'm in Thailand with Becca, and there was a flood," she

said calmly.

"Are you okay?" I asked groggily.

"Yes, but I'm at a hotel, and they told all the guests that we needed to call our families and tell them we're okay, so I did."

"That's great. I'm glad that you did."

"Bye, Mom. I have to go now, but I love you."

"Love you too. Bye."

I hung up the phone and went back to sleep.

I remembered Chelsea mentioning some sort of flood, so when I got up, I turned on the news. I was not worried because Chelsea had called to say the flood was over, and she was fine. I flipped on CNN.

Headline news: There had been a tsunami in Thailand, and Phuket had been destroyed.

The tsunami must have happened *after* I spoke to her, *after* the flood she spoke about. Where was my baby?!

All the phone lines were down, and the contact information she had given me was useless. I had no way to contact her. Braiden and Ty were at work. I was in a panic. I missed Alan more than ever. He was supposed to be here at times like this. What would he do?

I lay down on my bed, staring at the ceiling. "I need you now. I really need you," I cried.

But not for very long.

I had a daughter to find somewhere in Southeast Asia.

As in all crises, I phoned Jamie. She calmed me down and then suggested I call the parents of Chelsea's friend.

A man answered.

"This is Lynne Hanson, Chelsea Hanson's mom." I began

Where in the World Is Chelsea Hanson?

pacing, slowly, steadily. "I think that Chelsea and your daughter
are together in Thailand, Phuket to be exact, and I don't know
if you've heard, but there's been a tsunami there, and I was
hoping that you'd heard from them."

He had not.

How could he be so calm? Our daughters were in the
middle of a world disaster, and we could not find them! Yet he
was doing exactly what Alan would have done. Staying calm.
Maybe it is a man/woman thing.

"Let me give you some phone numbers, in case you can't
reach me." I rattled off the number to my cell phone, which
Braiden had insisted I buy, then Jamie's, Braiden's, and Ty's
cell numbers.

My baby was out there, lost in a disaster of epic proportions, and I had no idea if she was dead or alive. I had to keep
it together.

I phoned Braiden and Ty, and they phoned anyone who
might possibly have a connection to the latest news. We were
all in our own panic. I did not want to tell my mother or father
until we knew Chelsea was okay, which she would be, I told
myself.

All day, Jamie phoned. "Have you heard anything?"

"No, have you?"

"No."

Braiden phoned. "Have you heard anything?"

"No, have you?"

"No."

Ty phoned Braiden. "Have you heard anything?"

"No."

119

"Have you heard anything?"

"No."

Braiden phoned Jamie, "Have you heard anything?"

"No."

By now Karren had joined the chain.

After an excruciating twenty-four hours, Chelsea's friend's father called.

"They're okay. They're safe on an isolated island in the Gulf of Thailand. At the last minute they decided not to go to Phuket. They're okay." He sounded so relieved. He had hidden his fears well in the beginning.

Alan would have done that.

"Phone service is sporadic at best," he continued, "and they can't get off the island because all transportation has come to a complete stop. They're trying to get back to Bangkok, but it will take days, at least. I'll let you know if I hear anything, and please let me know if you hear anything."

When Chelsea was finally able to call, I sobbed unabashedly on the phone.

"I'm fine, Mom," she pleaded. "Remember, when I called earlier? I told you there was a flood."

Yes, she had.

It took her a week to get back to Bangkok. She had originally planned to travel to southern India, but that area had also been hit hard by the tsunami. Of course, she still wanted to go.

"Mom, believe me," she said. "It's safe to go to southern India. All my friends say it's safe."

"Prove it," I replied.

She tried, but in vain. She had a friend whose family lived

there, and her biggest mistake was asking the friend to email me: She only confirmed that it was not safe to go to southern India. Chelsea had to give in.

Instead, she spent a month traveling among the wonders of northern India. Poor baby. She continued to follow my contact rules, at one point emailing me what had to be my favorite contact instructions: If I needed to reach her, I should call Joe's Bar in a tiny town and ask someone to go about a mile down to the beach, turn left, travel past the cow, pig, and chicken, and she would be in the third hammock on the left.

That certainly gave me confidence.

She traveled to Dharamsala, the home of the exiled Dalai Lama, and was able to attend three weeks of teachings by the Dalai Lama himself.

"I'd love a photo of you with him," I said, much calmer now that she was out of the tsunami area.

"Haven't been able to do that," she replied. "But I got you some hats."

Hats would have to be good enough.

Chapter Twenty-Two

Is It My Turn?

ozeman's more "mature" populous seemed to consist of couples who hung out with other couples, or singles at bars. I was neither, so I spent even more time at home. Dating was the last thing on my mind. My body was the last thing on my mind.

I treated myself to a new dog, a Cavalier King Charles spaniel named Tula, but other than walks with Tula, my life was that of a hermit.

Braiden suggested we take a trip to Paris.

"I know this great hotel," she said, drumming her fingers on her thigh. "We call it Hotel One Star."

My parents had traveled all over the world, and my children had lived abroad many times, yet I had never been off this continent. It really was about time I did.

Hotel One Star was definitely named appropriately. The walls were stained, the bath was so cramped you could barely move, and the ceiling looked as if it would collapse at any minute. The staircase was steep and circular, and only about two feet wide, but each morning and evening we maneuvered it.

Lots of doctors were staying at the hotel, which I thought was a good sign. At least we would have medical attention if needed.

Our days were filled with walking the streets, visiting museums, sitting in parks, and people watching. For lunch we would buy crepes from a street vendor, and at night we would buy cheese and a baguette for about three dollars, then take our luxurious dinner back to our room and sit on our beds, eating and recounting the day.

The fashions of Paris were spectacular. Even though Braiden was much taller than most Parisians, her looks fit in with the svelte, sophisticated locals. She would pile her long dark hair loosely onto her head and layer odd pieces of clothes together in that sophisticated yet quirky way that Europeans do. Every day I was reminded that my wide potato body did not make the Parisian cut.

"That could be a good look for me, don't you think?" I would comment, looking at a chic outfit in a boutique window.

"That would be beautiful," Braiden would eagerly respond.

Then we would take a moment to picture me in those clothes. Not going to happen.

They needed breasts. Did I need breasts?

I tried scarves. Every woman in Paris wears a scarf.

I posed. "This look might work for me." It was half statement and half question.

"Scarves would be a great look for you! There are so many ways to wear one."

I purchased a few: two pashminas, one coral and one white, plus a spectacular multicolored one that was a total splurge. I loved the look but found that even the lightweight ones were hot and claustrophobic. Scarves were not going to save this body.

I bought a hat.

My body image was on a roller coaster, but I was not going to admit that to myself or anyone. One day I was proud of my boobless chest, and the next day, awkward and uncomfortable.

After we returned from Paris, I jumped at the opportunity to join a group of women on a trip to Portugal. Perfect! We would be a band of sisters, unconcerned about each other's bodies. I packed my baggy cargo pants, tees, and sweaters and had an incredible time making new friends and relishing the splendor of Portugal.

I bought a hat.

Next, it was off to Peru with Chelsea. It was a casual trip, so my clothes were not an issue. T-shirts were acceptable, and I ignored any discomfort with my booblessness, blissfully ignorant of how appalled I would be later when I saw my flat, two-dimensional body in the photos.

And I bought a hat.

Chapter Twenty-Three

Hello Good-bye

Chelsea and I had brought some of Alan's ashes with us to spread somewhere in Peru. The girls and I had been and still are spreading them around the world. He is in India, Kenya, and on his favorite surf beach in Santa Barbara, just to name a few places. Some day we will fly over the Grand Tetons in Wyoming, his favorite mountains, to spread more of him.

We decided to bring the ashes with us to the Machu Picchu graveyard, a flat area above the main part of the village ruins. We laid a small amount on the ground and closed our eyes to say a blessing. There was absolutely no wind whatsoever, just dead silence, but when we opened our eyes, the ashes were gone. No one said a word.

Chelsea and I needed time to be alone with our thoughts. I found a small ledge around the corner from the rest of the ruins, with about 3,000 feet of sheer granite cliff below it. I sat down as close to the granite wall as I could, away from the edge, and closed my eyes. A few moments later, when I opened them, five brightly colored parrots were flying right in front of me, no more than twenty feet away. They were as light and graceful as anything could be, in exquisite formation, without a crack in their perfect timing and spacing. I felt their beauty and freedom.

The Incas believed that odd numbers were good omens. I just knew that Alan was there and happy. I could feel him. Tears came, but not for my loss. I was sad, of course—my husband of thirty years was gone—but I was at peace knowing that his spirit, or whatever you want to call it, was there. He had always needed his nature fix, and he was deep inside it now. He was part of it.

That intense feeling of Alan actually being inside nature became a recurring incident. When Trent's mother visited from Australia, I took her to Yellowstone, but they were doing some roadwork along the drive into the park. It looked like we would be stopped there for a while.

"I'm going to get out and walk a bit," I told her, my voice uneasy.

She seemed to sense my need to be alone. "No worries," she replied.

We had stopped precisely at one of Alan's favorite fishing spots. I walked along the river until I was alone, and then felt Alan's presence deep in the water. The river was part of him, and he was part of the river. I had experienced this depth of feeling only once before, on the ledge in Machu Picchu, and for the first time since he had died, I began to sense that he was okay. All this time, I'd had an ever-present gnawing feeling that he was confused. Survivor's guilt lingers to this day. Why am I so lucky to still be with our girls and he's not? It's not logical to have this guilt, but it's so hard to shake. Now, alongside the river, alongside Alan, I realized that I wanted to be alive. I was here for a reason.

My father was not doing well. As he aged, the Parkinson's progressed, but we were able to reduce his medication. My mother and I were certain now that he had been in the study group that had received the stem cells. But this wouldn't be enough to save him.

He was nearing death. He knew it, and we knew it. His death was expected and planned for as well as it could be, so I was dealing with it in a completely different way than I had dealt with Alan's. My mother and Jamie came up immediately, but Lauren had already said her good-byes. We had the local rabbi come in to give my father his blessing.

He had donated his brain to the NIH/Columbia research study, which by now was at least twenty years old. I had been given specific instructions to follow, and it was time for me to make the arrangements. Trying not to think about what I was actually doing, I made the calls to DC and New York. The coordinator needed to talk to the doctor at the home, who needed to talk to the funeral home, who needed to talk to the coroner, who needed to talk to the doctor in charge of the program in New York. It was a complicated coordination, but it looked like we might be able to pull it off.

The study coordinator was a high-energy New Yorker, not accustomed to the laid-back accessibility that was common in a small town like Bozeman. "I've never talked to a coroner in his own home," she exclaimed in her thick New York accent.

"He said he would be honored to perform the procedure—as long as it didn't interfere with his skiing schedule."

That was Bozeman for you.

We were all able to be with Papa when he died, taking turns napping in a room the nurses gave us across the hall. He hung on all night, just to keep us up, I'm sure. I sat with him the entire time, holding his hand and telling him that everything was okay. He slept most of the time, only starting to wake up from discomfort when the medication wore off. I had some stupid movie on in his room, and when I was distracted by it for a moment, he let go. His breathing stopped. I called everyone into his room. He was gone.

My father, in charge until the end, had conveniently died at 5:30 a.m., just in time for the coroner to perform the procedure and get up to the mountain for the first run of the day. Papa would have not wanted the man to miss his skiing.

A few months later, the doctor in charge of the original stem cell study called both my mother and me. He was giddy with delight as he told us that my father had made history. The common belief had been that stem cells would not survive in the elderly population, but the tissue from my father's brain indicated that at the time of my his death, the cells were alive and well. The doctor sent us copies of his book just published on the subject, in which my father was referenced many times.

Chapter Twenty-Four

OMG, the Kentucky Derby!

I needed something to throw my grief into. I poured myself into my art and traveled extensively. Thinking that Tula needed a buddy when she was home alone, I found another cavalier, named Bennett.

From out of nowhere I received a phone call from a woman coordinating an art show in conjunction with the Kentucky Derby. Part of the show's proceeds would go to an organization that rescues ex-race horses. She had seen my artwork online, loved it, and tracked my work to one of the Montana galleries I was in.

I could not believe it. Little old me, showing my art at a Kentucky Derby show!

I decided to show some of my paintings, but I wanted to do something new for it as well, something unique that would combine my interests. The thought of getting my hands dirty really appealed to me, so I decided to sculpt a horse. I would make a basic sculpture, then use miniscule seed beads to cover the entire form and create a mixture of patterns and color.

Beading Braiden's skating dresses while I was recovering from my last mastectomy had been cathartic and fun. Perhaps I hoped it would be again, as I grieved the loss of another part of me, my father.

Then I faced the hardest task. I had to come up with some outfits to wear. The show was at the end of April, in Kentucky. Hot weather, hot receptions. I needed clothes that would keep me cool while looking hot. A bra and prostheses were not an option. I had grown comfortable without them and was afraid that wearing them would send me into a sweating stupor.

I had to look great. Not good, but great. This was going to be ten times harder than creating the artwork.

I had to create me.

Bozeman is hardly the shopping capital of the world, so I went online. Orders from everywhere arrived on my doorstep.

"This pile is from Nordies, this is from Macy's, this is from Breton, and this one is from Anthropologie," I explained to Ty, Braiden, and Chelsea.

I would carefully fold each discarded top into its respective return pile.

"I like this one from Anthro." Braiden held up the next top for me to try on, and then all three would vote on which ones they liked. They were having a blast, but I was in hell. Trying on clothes in front of three fashionistas was daunting at best, but with only a tank top to protect their fragile eyes from my scarred chest, it was a lesson in humility. I chose some pieces that had pleated detailing to cover my flat top. They would do.

It ended up being a fairy tale trip. I had been to Kentucky to do some art fairs, but this one was huge. Gail still lived in Kentucky, so she joined me. My work got rave reviews.

I felt like my life was on track, but my body image was not keeping up with the pace.

Chapter Twenty-Five

Rowena

*J*ust as I was thinking that our lives had settled into a smooth rhythm, Braiden decided to go to grad school in art history. She got accepted at the University of Maryland and was off to DC, where I had grown up. At the same time, and equally unexpected, Chelsea applied to law school and was accepted to one in St. Paul, Minnesota. After all her travels, I was worried that she would be bored in a such a calm place. But the rigors of law school took care of that. Then, of course, Ty returned to New York City.

I was alone.

The house was empty, and I needed a buddy, so I decided to sculpt one. Why not? She would be about four feet tall, with her arms spread wide, dancing. Back in my sweatshirt designing days, I had drawn a wonderful fat dancing ballerina, and my buddy would be made in her likeness. I would put her in my bedroom. She could wear my hats.

The only human sculpture I had ever done was that awful head back in Seattle, but I was not worried. I could do it if I just set my mind to it. Of course, it did not hurt that Jamie was a skilled sculptor.

I called her from Home Depot. "Hey, it's me." When together, we loved to wander its wide aisles to find inspiration and materials, and Jamie was an artistic MacGyver. She could figure out how to make anything. I didn't see any reason she couldn't do the same over the phone. And I was right.

"I need to find something to make the base of the body with."

"Use the cardboard tubing that's used to make concrete columns," she replied without hesitation.

That was the first of many such calls, and Jamie had all the answers. As I usually talk with my hands, I could be seen meandering down aisles, seemingly talking to myself, and collecting a most unusual assortment of materials.

The sculpture began with a two-foot-diameter cardboard tube. Added to that was chicken wire, which formed her torso. Her arms were PVC pipes and her head, crushed up aluminum foil, clay, and other miscellaneous items. Rocks from the back yard stabilized her.

"I need something to make the arms rigid."

"Find a medical supply store and buy the rolls of fiberglass that are used for casts."

I found lime green fiberglass at a huge discount. Not skilled in the art of wrapping casts, I never even considered that it might be a good idea to wear gloves. A layer of fiberglass adhered to my hands, making them lime green for days, but the casting material worked beautifully, allowing her to extend her arms in glee.

I covered the mishmash of materials with layers upon layers of plaster cast material and fabric. Somewhere along the line, my short ballerina grew to be my tall, wide ballerina. She ended up about five and a half feet tall and four feet wide. And flat. Flat as a board.

I painted a black leotard and ballet slippers on her. She was tiptoed, head cocked just so, to show her delight with the world. Her hair was painted on her head in a tight bun.

I named her Rowena, after a housekeeper we'd had when I was a child. She would rub alcohol on my back when I was sick, and it had always made me feel better.

Chapter Twenty-Six

Signs

*R*owena and I were doing well, but as the temperature increased, so did my anxiety. Summer was art fair season, which meant once again facing my clothing dilemma. It was important that I dress as a serious artist, which meant both professional and artsy, but also that I be able to do the physical work required to set up and dismantle my booth in the heat of summer, which meant staying as cool as possible. I began to dread shows because I had to figure out what to wear. Stupid, I know, but it was that important to me.

There had to be other women with this problem. I was a clothing designer and could not work with the clothes available in stores—others must have been having an even more difficult time.

The idea of a clothing line lingered in the back of my mind. My art career was going well despite the sinking economy, yet I could feel something calling to me. I am always looking for connections in life and positive reasons for things happening the way they do. I am a percolator, just like the old-fashioned one with the glass top that my mother made coffee in when I was growing up. I loved watching the water turn from clear to a rich deep brown while listening to the noise the coffee made as it popped up into the glass.

Thoughts, ideas, experiences, and feelings had been percolating inside me. When I had first felt Alan's presence in the river, I had realized I was still here for a reason. Now I was beginning to wonder if that reason, and the reason for the cancer, the mastectomies, the problems with the implant, the clothing struggles—all of it—was so I could design a clothing line for women like me.

Since my mastectomies, now fifteen years ago, I had fought the battle to be flat. I was determined that I did not need breasts. After all, my breasts had been so small from the start, and I had always hated wearing a bra. At this point in a woman's life, her breasts become saggy anyway, more of a nuisance than an asset. I was not interested in dating, so I did not need them for a man. I did not need them for breastfeeding. I did not need them. Or want them. But I did want to look good. I wanted to look like a three-dimensional, feminine woman.

I thought, no, I *knew* without hesitation that there must be other women like me, who have had mastectomies or who were naturally flat. They still wanted to be feminine. I was a clothing designer, for God's sakes! I could create this! Nothing had ever seemed clearer to me. The signs were all there. The newspapers seemed filled with stories of celebrities having mastectomies. Another sign. Choosing mastectomies without reconstruction was a growing trend.

Women all over were facing the challenge of losing what our society defines as their femininity. My mission would be to help them feel confident and beautiful no matter what shape or lack of shape their cancer had left their breasts in. Oprah would embrace me as the one who had changed everything. All of womankind would applaud me for liberating them.

I even had the perfect name for the line: Annie Flats! This was why that name was in my life, and why it had been so important for me to keep it when I bought out my partner. Back then, I had assumed it mattered because it was a family name, but now I was certain that I had been emphatic about it so that I would have it for this moment. I had resigned myself to being boring Lynne, but now, maybe I had an opportunity to be Annie again. Annie would be back in business, and so would Flats.

My idea was twofold. First, I would design the clothes with the specific needs of women like me in mind. I would use myself as both market and fit model. If I would wear it, it would work. It was so easy! The premise behind the designs was to use fabrics and detailing to confuse the eye, so that what was actually beneath the clothes would be vague.

Second, I would launch a campaign to educate women on "going flat," or "natural," as a positive alternative to dangerous implants or uncomfortable prostheses. Annie Flats would send a message of strength, confidence, and beauty. I am not sure whom I was trying to convince, other people or myself, but it did not matter. This campaign would become my life obsession.

This was my noble cause. I would be the Mother Teresa of breasts.

One minor problem. Sewing. My blood pressure would go sky high when I sat in front of a sewing machine. I had been a good patternmaker in my day, and I knew how to sew, but my craftsmanship was terrible. I needed my priceless creations to be perfect. I needed to find help. But try as I might, that help was not materializing in Bozeman.

This only contributed to a growing uneasiness with my life. Although I adored Bozeman and the house I had worked so hard to stay in and finish, I was alone. Rowena just was not doing it for me. Bozeman seemed to be a town of couples and young adventurers. I was neither. Well, maybe an old adventurer.

I clicked with one woman, Birdie, who coincidentally was from DC, not far from where I had grown up. Her daughter was attending graduate school in Bozeman, so her family had purchased a vacation home there. Whenever she was in town, we would explore garage sales together, and whenever I was in DC visiting Braiden, we would make time to get together.

Even so, I was a hermit, concentrating on my artwork and planning my clothing line. Days would go by without my seeing anyone, and in the back of my mind was the knowledge that Alan had died alone and the uneasy thought that if something were to happen to me, no one would find me.

I got into the habit of calling Jamie first thing every morning.

"Still alive" was the only thing I needed to say.

Someone needs to know that I am still breathing.

Finally, I decided to move to Colorado Springs, where Jamie had her ranch. I needed her now, and I liked to think that she needed me—as family, as a friend, as a yak herder. Yes, she had added yaks to her assortment..

In Colorado, I could work on my line and be safe. I still loved Bozeman and did not want to give up the dream completely, so I would try to hang on to the house. As an added bonus, Colorado Springs had a world-class ice-skating program. I would find my patternmakers and sample sewers from the many skating costume makers there.

Another sign!

Chapter Twenty-Seven

The Next Leap

On an early April morning, I left Bozeman. It had been five years since Alan and I had arrived there to live out our dream. The movers had packed up Rowena and my belongings and were on their way. I packed the most fragile of my possessions into my car and headed off with Tula, Bennett, and Mona Soup. I was a veteran of road trips. I had my pretzel rods, twenty-ounce bottle of Pepsi, and stock traveling music—with the addition of the soundtrack to *Shall We Dance*.

It was snowing lightly, but the forecast had not mentioned anything unusual. In Montana, only a raging snowstorm, if that, would stop you. Two hours into the trip, it started snowing harder, and within four hours, it was a blizzard. I stopped in Sheridan, Wyoming, to get gas and found out that all roads and highways had closed. I was stranded.

There was a long line in the lobby of the Super 8. People were friendly, but apprehensive. All of us needed a place to stay, and there were only a finite number of hotel rooms available.

"Which way are you going?" asked the guy in front of me,

a tall, burly man in a Fed Ex uniform.

"South," I replied. "But not today. Which way are you going?"

"North. I'm driving that huge truck out there in the parking lot." He gestured toward the lobby window. I could barely make out the shadow of a large Fed Ex truck. The snow and wind had picked up considerably. I thought of my little SUV, packed to the brim, with two dogs and a cat waiting inside, and hoped it wasn't buried already.

"Fed Ex reserved a room for me, but now they're telling me to keep driving," he said. "I don't know if they realize how bad it is, but corporate says to drive, so I'm going. I was just standing in line to give it up, but if you'd like, I'll give it to you."

Wow, what luck!

"I'd love that! Thank you so much. And if you do have to turn around, I'll be happy to share it with you." That was the least I could do, and only fair, I thought. This man seemed like a harmless gentle giant. I'd take my chances.

The front desk clerk announced that all rooms were booked, so the driver and I stepped forward, and I was given his room.

I smuggled the pets into my room through the back door. I didn't want to take the chance of asking if I could bring them in. If the clerk said no, I couldn't leave them in the car to freeze, and every other hotel in town was booked. I had been planning on making the trip in one day, so I'd brought no provisions for Mona. I had to take my life into my hands and drive to the K-mart a few doors down to pick up some cat food, kitty litter, and an aluminum baking pan for a kitty litter tray. By the skin of my teeth, I made it back to the hotel, sort of walked the dogs, and settled in for what I thought would be one night.

Boy, was I wrong. The snow didn't stop. The roads didn't open. In the midst of the next big leap in my life, I was suddenly frozen in midair.

My Fed Ex guy had been turned around and was back at the hotel. Somehow he had been able to get a room. I lined up with the other guests to rebook my room, and when some mentioned that the Subway was open, a bunch of us headed out to scrape the snow and ice off our cars and try to navigate the snow-packed, icy local streets.

The Fed Ex man was sitting in his truck, eating a sandwich and reading. "Have you found the Subway?" I asked.

"No, I can't drive this big rig around the city streets," he said. "I walked over to the gas station across the street." He motioned toward a blank sheet of snow. "They had some prepackaged sandwiches, but they're running out."

"I think I can get out," I said. "Why don't you come with me?"

"Sure, sounds great." He jumped out of his truck, locked it up with the gentleness of a father with his baby, and we headed toward my car. He had to contort himself to fit into the passenger seat.

The narrow city streets were lined with piles of snow, abandoned cars, parked cars, and fallen tree branches. The snow was coming down hard, and my windshield wipers were having trouble keeping up. We had to keep stopping to wipe away the heaps of snow weighing them down. Every time, after he got out to wipe away the snow, my gentle giant had to figure out how to get back in, trying new ways of squishing his large, wet body into the seat.

The sandwiches were delicious, but after three days of this, Subway got a bit old. Each day, we would line up to rebook our rooms as we found out that the roads were closed for yet another day.

The dogs needed to be walked, but the snow had piled up several feet higher than they were, so it was a precarious and short adventure out of the room. A few other people had pets, but we kept them in our rooms and quiet. As we walked through the halls, we would nod to each other knowingly.

I was running out of food for the animals, having bought the smallest possible bags at K-mart that first day, thinking we'd be in Colorado the next, so my Fed Ex buddy and I headed over to the grocery store across from the Subway after lunch, walking in to the most bizarre sight. The entire store was just about empty, and I'm not talking about people. There was hardly any stock. Delivery trucks had been unable to get through, yet the town was full of trapped travelers, like an isolated, overpopulated island. I spotted some dog and cat food left, and it was like I'd hit the mother lode.

The movers had left ahead of the storm and made it to Colorado Springs. While watching *Judge Judy* on my hotel bed, with two restless dogs and one confused cat jumping around me, I directed Jamie in placing my furniture.

"Have them put the red hutch in the living room, which is going to become my studio. I want it by the fireplace."

"It doesn't fit next to the fireplace," said Jamie. "It's about three inches too big."

"Okay, let's try the wall across from the fireplace. Tula, stop terrorizing Mona! Try Rowena by the picture window. She'll enjoy the view."

"Call you back."

Finally, on the fourth day, the interstate opened. In my life, when something starts out bad, it ends up great. If this strange luck still applied, my new life was going to be amazing.

Jamie had set up my new town home beautifully. The large living room (now studio) had vaulted ceilings, a fireplace, and a magnificent view of the mountains, with southern light filling the room. An indestructible floor cloth that Braiden and I had made covered the pecan-stained wood floors. Two dining tables pushed together made one huge work table. The red hutch held my art supplies, and I found two ornate, boudoir-looking chandeliers that filled the room with even more light. Rowena moved from window to window, confusing passersby as to what or who she was.

The dining room was now my living room. French doors led to a patio, where I would spend my evenings percolating plans for my new life while looking out on the mountains.

Tula, Mona, and I adjusted well, but Bennett was not happy. She fell in love with my neighbor's grandson, who was visiting from Boston, and not one to want an unhappy dog, I let her move to Boston. Tula and Mona were thrilled.

I signed up for dance lessons. Ballroom dance. It was on my bucket list, and I was on a roll. This was going to be tricky, however; I worried when someone hugged or held me that they were wondering where the boobs were. Where the bra strap was.

But I was just going to have to get over it and dance.

The lessons were fun, but I felt like a pathetic old deformed lady who had to pay a gigolo to be with her. I valiantly attended the "socials," where the few male dancers would make the rounds, dancing with the women without partners.

Women without partners—sounds like a support group.

I pushed myself to go to a dance seminar. I marched into the studio, proud of myself, sticking out my chest to show the world that I was woman.

"You, in the brown shirt," the instructor twanged. "Hon, come on over here and show everyone what *not* to do with their posture. You're doing it so well."

It has been a while since I have taken dance lessons.

Chapter Twenty-Eight

Women without Partners

One day, while I was visiting Chelsea and we were out walking the beautiful city streets near her law school, she blurted out, "Mom, you need to start dating." I could tell that she had been working up the nerve to say this, and it had just come out with the intensity only Chelsea could muster.

Life with Chelsea was always a statement, not a question.

She was never one to mince words, or to talk just for the sake of talking, so the silence that followed was not unexpected.

Then: "Dad's been gone for a while now, and I think it's time for you to date."

More silence.

"Why do I have to date?"

"You need new friends and need to get out and do things."

"I have friends, and I do things."

"But you need to date."

"I'll think about it. I love you."

I wasn't interested in dating, but maybe I would give

dancing another try if I could find someone to dance with. I decided to try to find my dancing soul mate.

I signed up for J-Date, an Internet dating service for Jews. I figured that we'd have something in common, being Jewish, and by going with the dating service, it wouldn't put pressure on friends to find dates for me. If it didn't work out, there wouldn't be any hard feelings. Perfect.

So I signed up and let the service find my perfect matches. First one—a woman in her sixties. Whoops. I'm pretty sure that I'm not a lesbian, but maybe the Internet knew something I didn't. Besides, I was only fifty-eight. Why couldn't I go out with some young chick? My experiences with Internet dating never did include a date with another woman, but there were many, many, too many disastrous first dates.

One man seemed very nice—intelligent and not bad looking. We emailed a few times; then I let him phone me. We chatted a bit. He had two dogs that he loved, and as Karren had told me, any man I dated had to have a pet and had to have kids, so he seemed like a good candidate. We set up a meeting at a park not far from my house. We would bring the dogs, let them play at the park, and then go out for lunch. This sounded safe enough.

First red flag. He kept telling me that he was going to bring me flowers. Well, I love flowers as much as anyone, but let's not think that flowers will conquer the world. Or the woman.

It was important to me not to hide my flatness. I didn't want to flaunt it in his face, but I didn't want to hide it either. Luckily, it was spring, so I could pretty much wear whatever I wanted. Since we were going to a park, I dressed in my comfortable-yet-not-sweats cargo pants and largish cashmere sweater, with a t-shirt under it. This was my Colorado dressed-up outfit. Going on a date was already way out of my comfort zone, so dressing comfortably was crucial to me.

I arrived at the park a bit early and let Tula off her leash to play fetch with her ball. Not long after I arrived, I saw a small man walking toward me with an adorable dog and a very sorry, crumpled, dying bunch of flowers wrapped in an old plastic grocery bag. The flowers looked like they'd come from some-one's garbage bag, but hey, he was nice enough to bring flowers, so I'd give him a chance.

"Do you like the flowers? See, I brought you flowers, what do you think of them? I told you I'd bring you flowers, and look, here they are. Just as I said I'd do. What do you think of them?"

I was speechless.

"Thank you so much. They're very pretty," I responded politely.

"Here, take the flowers. I told you I'd bring you flowers, and here they are. What do you think of them?" He insisted. He was a journalist, so maybe he was just trained to get to the truth. But that was the last thing I was going to tell him.

"They're very nice. Thank you so much," I responded as he shoved them in my face.

I put Tula's leash down and took the old wrinkled grocery bag with the wilted flowers. They were past their glory days and were begging to be composted.

"Your dog is so pretty. What's her name?" I asked.

"Mandy." Period.

"How old is she?"

"Seven." Period.

"My dog is five."

Silence.

"What exactly do you do for a living?" was the next question that came to my mind.

"I'm a journalist." Period.

This conversation wasn't going anywhere, and neither was this date. I asked a few more questions and then decided that I was sick of this game, and we threw the ball for the dogs in dead silence.

"Shall we go get lunch?" I asked. "I saw a nice restaurant with outdoor tables around the corner, so we can take the dogs there."

"Yes. We can put your flowers right in the middle of the table." Well, at least I got a few more words out of him. He must be a lousy journalist, I thought. Or maybe he's a good one, the way he just picks one topic and obsesses about it until you're worn down.

We walked a few short blocks to the restaurant and found a nice table. It was small, and the tables were close to the other guests, but it was quaint.

"Put your flowers right here, right in the middle of the table." I had placed them at my side, because there was no room on the table, but I put the floppy flowers right smack in the middle. Happy?

Each of us ordered lunch, and the waitress could do nothing right.

She came out with glasses of water and some bread and

butter. There was no room, so I moved the grocery bag toward me, and she wiggled the glasses and bread bowl onto the table.

"I want more ice in my water," he demanded. My pet peeve is when people don't say please and thank you. At first he was just harmless and annoying, but now I was starting to fume.

"I don't like that type of bread. I want another type," he continued to quibble.

"The salad has too much dressing on it. The sandwich is too hot. Do you like the flowers, aren't they beautiful? What do you think of the flowers? Where are you going to put the flowers when you get home? Aren't they beautiful? Well, what do you think of me? Do you like me? What are we going to do next?"

I took a deep breath and couldn't look him in the eye. I looked down at Tula and his dog, who had been dutifully sitting by our sides, waiting for a crumb to fall.

"You seem very nice," I stuttered.

"Honestly, you can tell me. What do you think of me? You can be honest. Tell me."

"I just don't think we have anything in common" was the nastiest I could get. I expected him to continue to question me about him, or to at least ask me how I liked the flowers, but instead he jumped out of his chair, jerking his poor dog up by the collar. She flew through the air as he knocked his chair over.

"Well, I guess I'm just an asshole," he yelled as he ran out of the table area. He was across the street and into a car before I could even start to comprehend what had just happened. I was speechless. The customers eating next to us stared at me with disbelief. What in the world had just happened? I was shaking. Luckily, we had already paid (we'd split the bill), so I tried to collect myself, grabbing the sorry flowers for some reason, and with a confused Tula, shakily walked home. This was a good one for the book of why Lynne doesn't want to date.

Sorry, Chelsea.

Chapter Twenty-Nine

Patience, Prudence

I had better luck meeting new friends than meeting dance partners. I met Carolyn when I volunteered at a local ice-skating competition, and we became instant walking buddies. It was an unlikely match. She, the epitome of class and elegance, was always dressed immaculately, her hair coifed, with perfect makeup, and I was usually wearing my baggy cargo pants and faded cashmere sweater, with a bit of makeup here and there.

I came into her life as she was losing her husband to a prolonged illness. I seemed to be what she needed at the time, as she was what I needed. Our backgrounds were as different as night and day, but we were connected from the start. I have found in my many moves that the people who come into our lives are there for a reason. The reason might be for them or for me—it didn't matter, and I couldn't tell you which one of us needed the other. Probably both.

I met another friend on one of my walks. One day Tula and I were strolling down a lovely street when a car drove by, stopped, and started backing up. The driver was about my age, and she looked sane, even though she was excitedly waving her arms at me.

"I have the same type of dog as you!" she exclaimed.

You have to understand that Tula's breed was not a normal western mountain dog. She was the only cavalier in Bozeman and was a sight hiking with the labs and retrievers along the rugged Montana trails. Seeing another cavalier, especially in the mountains, is like seeing a long lost friend. The lady introduced herself as Linda, and her dog was Lucy. We chatted for a while on the side of the street, and she invited us to her home, around the corner. Lucy and Tula greeted each other with the comfort of old cousins, and we spent the next hours with our new buds. After that, every Monday we met and had great walks with our dogs. Tula developed a girl crush on Lucy and knew the way to her house from ours. I think if she ever got lost, she would go to Lucy's before mine.

Linda owned a shoe and accessory store downtown, called Saboz. She had lived in Colorado for many years and was well connected with the businesses in town. She was eager to help me find a sample maker. Linda introduced me to Jan, who owned a small jacket company called Janska. They made jackets for people who were disabled, such as those confined to a wheelchair, as well as people going through chemotherapy. The jackets were well thought out and made of a practical and warm fabric called Polartec.

Jan and I were interested in each other's concepts. She did not know of anyone who could help me, but she asked if I would be interested in helping her take her line to a more fashion-forward place, because they were looking to get into more upscale boutiques. Fantastic. I could use the money, and their connections would help me with my line. I had always been the type of person who needed to have things done yesterday, but this time I was going to be different and let things happen organically. Patience would be my new mantra.

Little did I know that both Jamie and I were about to be taught a new lesson in patience.

One day, as I was about to leave my house to meet an old skating friend who was in town for a competition, Jamie called. "I need you," she said frantically.

"What's up? I'm about to leave for lunch," I said, a bit annoyed. She knew I had been looking forward to seeing my old friend.

"The yaks have escaped."

Yaks, I have learned, are nasty creatures. Jamie had needed some animals to put on her property in the mountains, and yaks didn't require much attention (or so she had thought). Plus, she could sell their hair for weaving. Jamie never does anything lightly, so instead of getting one or two yaks, she got eight. And one was pregnant. Yaks are not nice at any time, but especially not when pregnant or when they have a baby. And did I mention that they have pointed horns that extend at least a foot out of their skulls? I kept bugging Jamie to put tennis balls on the ends of the horns to make them a bit safer, but she never even got close enough to try. They are strange creatures; they look like a horse, cow, pig, and longhorn all rolled up into one odd ball.

"Where did they go?"

"We think they are near a neighbor's ranch."

The neighbor had called a neighbor who had called a neighbor when he woke up and saw eight yaks outside his front window. Not a normal sight in the Rocky Mountains.

"We need to go up there and try to catch them or something."

"Something" being the operative word. The yaks were not about to let someone catch them.

I sighed and rubbed the bridge of my nose. "I'll cancel my lunch and be ready to go."

We found them grazing near the horses on a neighbor's ranch. On one side of them was a fence with a small gate, and on the other three sides was nothing but land. They were free to go absolutely anywhere in the vast Rocky Mountains. This was going to be a challenge. There were seven of us—including Jamie, me, my nephew's girlfriend, Jamie's other ranch hand, and the neighbor up in the mountains—trying to catch eight nasty, aggressive thousand-pound beasts. This would work.

We decided to try somehow to round the yaks toward the gate, where we'd made a small pen out of portable metal fence piping. We latched the sections of fencing together so that if by some miraculous chance we were able to get the yaks into the pen, we could take out sections to make it smaller and smaller, forcing the yaks into Jamie's horse trailer, which was parked with the back ramp open at the gate. This was a great plan with one major flaw. How in the world would we get all the yaks, at one time, into the pen?

Most of us were on foot. The neighbors had two all-terrain vehicles. The plan was for us to try to get behind them and slowly come forward to push them toward the pen. In the pen was lots of hay to tempt them. The grass wasn't that good, so hopefully they would be hungry and smell the hay. We had to get way beyond the yaks to get around them, because they could run away from the pen at any time they felt threatened. Slowly, very slowly, we moved in. We had at least 500 yards between us, so it would have been easy for any of the yaks to take off away from the pen, and we would have never seen them again.

But somehow, it worked. It took a long time, but we were patient, and the yaks were hungry. We were able to get them into the pen, and slowly, as they calmed down, we would carefully remove a section of the fence. There was even more hay in the trailer, and for some joyous reason, they all went peacefully into it. We quickly closed the gate to the trailer, and thanked the neighbors profusely for their help. One of them commented about it being nice to meet Jamie's big sister, which I didn't bother to correct because one, we were in a hurry to get the trailer of yaks back to Jamie's ranch, and two, I was getting used to it. I had a couple of inches on Jamie and way more than a couple of gray hairs. Her wavy brown hair seemed to be just barely starting to gray. Everyone assumed she was younger than I was.

Jamie didn't keep the yaks longer. She had finally met her match. And I added yak herding to my resume.

With helping Jamie on her ranch and continuing to work on Janska's line, I hadn't done anything with mine. It was time to get on with my mission.

I had not yet found my perfect patternmaker, so I decided it was time to do some patternmaking of my own. After all, I used to work as one, albeit thirty-five years ago, but I was good at it then, and I could be good at it now.

I bought a dress form to drape the pattern from and began the surgical procedure. It was crucial that the dress form have the same body as I did. The more I cut, the more cathartic the process became. I was cutting away the grief of losing my breasts, the grief of losing my husband, the grief of losing the life we had dreamed of for over thirty years.

What I had cut away exposed the inner body. Me exposed—to the air, to the world, to myself. It was important to close me up quickly. I began to reconstruct. At first I used strips of fabric and plaster, which covered the expanse. I bought every type of bandage and fabric I could find to remake me and experimented with combinations of bandages, plaster, and fabrics until I found the perfect solution. I measured and remeasured every inch of the form until it matched my own. It was tedious and emotional, but the mannequin had to reflect reality. Finally, with an old form-fitting T-shirt covering the torso, voilà! Me. My deformed dress form was ready to be transformed into a beautiful woman. My designs would do that for her. For me.

I tried purchasing ready-made patterns from the fabric stores, hoping to simply alter them for my purposes. Much to my disappointment, they did not work. The disfigured body of a mastectomy patient was different from a breast-toting body, even a tiny-breasted breast-toting body. Fabrics draped differently. It did not make sense, but my dress form proved it true. I drew, draped, drafted, and pulled out old patternmaking books.

I even sewed.

Chapter Thirty

Vamoose

While struggling with the patterns, I needed to find "the" wonder fabric that could hold a shape while still being soft and natural, cool yet warm.

New York was the place to go.

In New York, I would search for my fabric, meet with potential resources for Janska, attend Ty's ice-skating show, and see family. Then I would head down to DC to see Braiden and her boyfriend, Ben. It looked like a serious relationship; they were talking about moving in with each other.

I love New York. As a naive "starving" art student, it had been tough, but now I embraced the vibrancy of the city. I wandered the streets of the garment district, in awe of the endless aisles of fabrics from around the world. Within hours, I found my wonder fabric. This was so easy, it was meant to be! Another sign. The fabric was made from bamboo, soft and cool for those of us still dealing with hot flashes and a sustainable "green" fabric to boot. Perfect. I bought a few yards and held my dreams in my arms.

Then I met with Remi, a potential resource for Janska. China was the place to have garments manufactured inexpensively, but there could be many complications, so they were looking for a middleman they could trust.

"Trust me," Remi kept saying. "I can make anything happen for you." The repetition got old.

In the end, Janska stuck to their grassroots program and continued to manufacture in the United States.

Next was Anders, a gregarious gentleman in his late forties. Janska had asked him to show me around to find new fabrics. We explored the small tucked-away offices of fabric resellers. He loved talking to everyone, wandering off subject, having a grand old time. It was fun, but not productive. I had already seen most of the fabrics on my own and was anxious to move on.

When in New York I treat myself to two very special meals. The first is at a hole-in-the-wall Chinese restaurant that makes the most incredible soup dumplings I've ever tasted. I could live on them. The other is a corned beef sandwich from Carnegie Deli. Yes, it is touristy and fatty, but a treat. I got a sandwich to eat on my bus ride to DC.

The buses from New York to DC are inexpensive and can be sketchy. One of the first was the "Downtown" bus, which was known for its irregular schedules, breakdowns on the New Jersey Turnpike, and drug busts. New bus lines were popping up all the time, and I booked a seat on one of them, Vamoose.

Sandwich in hand, I was welcomed at the bus door by the driver, John from Russia.

"Free soda for all students," John greeted everyone in his heavy Russian accent. "You need the caffeine to study. Not a student? Here, have a soda anyway."

From the outside, the bus resembled a rock star's traveling machine, right down to the black-tinted windows. I sat in a row by myself, three rows behind the driver's seat.

John continued to hand out sodas to the students, whose study habits concerned him. I loved John. I loved this bus. I had never been happier.

"What movie would all of you like?" John asked enthusiastically. "We have *The Gladiator* or *My Big Fat Greek Wedding.* You want *Big Fat Greek Wedding*? Good. That's the one I want too."

As the bus got rolling, I settled in for my adventure with an unobstructed view of the little TV screen above John. We passed the disgusting oil refineries, then got on the New Jersey Turnpike. Poor New Jersey. It gets a bum rap. It's actually a beautiful state, but not many people get beyond the initial yuck to see how lovely the rest of it is. Maybe that was for the best; it might stay beautiful.

I was feeling content, almost elated. I had found my wonder fabric, had seen family in New York, was heading to see Braiden and Ben, and was eating a Carnegie Deli sandwich while watching *My Big Fat Greek Wedding.* What could be better?

I was engrossed in the movie when the bus pulled over to the shoulder of the left lane. The turnpike was now a four-lane road with only a three-foot-tall cement barricade between us and the masses of oncoming cars. John got out of the bus. Was it Vamoose's turn to have the same fate as the Downtown bus? We waited in silence.

Then John returned to the bus. "My glasses blew out the draft window." He got in his seat, closed the door to the bus, and started backing up, on the left shoulder, with lots of oncoming traffic—and without his glasses.

This is the end. I am going to die. But I can't die. I have breastless women to save!

He stopped the bus again and got out. Either we would die or John would, and we would be stuck here for eternity.

Then he was back, waving the glasses and smiling ear to ear. They were intact! He fastened his seatbelt and off we went.

The bus was silent.

Chapter Thirty-One

With a Little Help from the Pros

DC was fun, Ben got my seal of approval, and I returned to Colorado Springs ready to leap into my obsession.

Linda introduced me to Gabrielle, my savior.

She arrived in a huge Cadillac. Joan of Arc in a Cadillac. She was in her seventies but looked younger, had bright red coiffed hair and flawless makeup. Maybe too much makeup and too colorful, but perfectly applied. She wore tight-fitting clothes in bright colors and lots of matched jewelry. Her heavy French accent completed the package.

I had donned my favorite baggy cargo pants, a form-fitting tank top, and the oversized pink shirt that used to house my hamster. No makeup. I was going to be the serious artist, too busy to worry about my looks.

"I'm a breast cancer survivor, and I want to produce a line of clothes for women who have had mastectomies and don't want or can't have reconstruction and just want to be flat." My spiel was well rehearsed by now.

Dead silence. Gabrielle, with her femininity oozing, looked at me blankly.

"Why do you want to design these clothes?" she asked, her accent coming through in long *eee's* and *z's* in place of *s's*. "I don't understand. Why would you not want the breasts?"

Then, after a moment, she said, "Okay, . . ." and flapped her hands against her hips. "Whatever you want." She would do this, but with an arrogant French flair.

Why in the world would I not want breasts? Having these spectacular objects is part of being a woman. And why would anyone want to wear loose clothes? My drab lumpy body looked ridiculous next to her bright pink knit top and equally bright green pants, hugging her curves.

I took control. "Why don't we start by making a basic pattern?"

"Whatever you wish," she said aloofly.

I handed her a tape measure and removed my blouse to have her take measurements. *Keep up the front,* I told myself. *Stay in control.* I wanted to die. I'd had a safe life until now, hiding my damaged torso under baggy sweatshirts, overalls, and potato sack dresses, but to make this obsession of mine work, it was necessary for me to expose my scars.

"My measurements are important," I said in an authoritarian way to hide my humiliation. "Because after a mastectomy, your body is different from someone who just has small breasts. More body mass has been taken away, so the proportion of the back to front is different than a normal pattern."

Wow, that sounded good.

"Okay." Her face was still blank. I had her take precise measurements of my chest, up and down, around and through. If I had to do this, I might as well do it right and get it over with. The patterns had to fit me perfectly, since I would be the guinea pig for the line.

A week later, she had the pattern and first muslin ready for fitting. This time I would go to her house. She lived in an area of small cottage-like homes. The Cadillac, which was proportionally too large for the row of white cottages, was parked along the street. Her front yard was landscaped with a few flowering plants. I knocked instead of trying the old-fashioned doorbell, and a dog went into a barking frenzy. Gabrielle came to the door with a small black poodle, which was still barking.

"Hellooooo. Come in."

Mahogany paneling, which looked like the house's original woodwork, lined the walls. Knickknacks, china teacups, porcelain figurines, and small paintings filled the rooms. It was a lovely home. It fit her. Everything was delicate. The house and her stuff had definitely seen better days, but you could tell that everything in the house was important to her, representing years of collecting with her now-deceased husband and reminders of her children and grandchildren.

She led me into a small sunroom, where she proudly showed me the area she had created for our projects. This was a promising sign. I just hoped she was good.

She was. We created our first masterpieces.

My first disciple, Nina, was a friend who'd had a single mastectomy. One aspect of my designs was to enable single-mastectomy women to shun prostheses. I had watched her fumble with her migrating prosthesis, discreetly trying to shove it back into place. Who would not want to throw away that plastic, anatomically correct weighted blob?

Nina had been intrigued by my line. "It's beautiful!" She was always so enthusiastic. My first creation would go to her.

I was not ready to use my precious bamboo fabric but instead found a gorgeous coral knit. From a slightly scooped banded neckline, strategically placed folds of fabric draped down to hide the fact that she was lopsided.

"Love it, love it, love it!" Nina raved as she twirled around, admiring herself in the mirror.

"Why don't you take it home, wear it, and see how you feel." I was beaming.

"I'd love to!" There was no hesitation in her voice. She felt good.

"Please let me know how you wear it and how you feel. That will help me a lot."

I would learn from her.

At first she was uncomfortable wearing it in public without a prosthesis, but gradually she became more comfortable, and I could see her transformation before my eyes.

My mission took hold of me.

Gabrielle and I continued. This was not a full-time obsession for her, so I kept my eyes open for another sewer to add to the team, now using an abbreviated spiel: "Hi, my name is Lynne Hanson, and I'm creating a clothing line for breast cancer survivors who have chosen not to wear or can't wear a prosthesis or have an implant."

I was usually greeted with silence or a quick response that told me they were not listening: "We can do anything you want. Just trust us."

Next.

This was a tough sell, to explain what my goal was, what fit I needed. How could they understand? After all, they had not undergone a mastectomy, lived flat chested, and performed a mastectomy on a dress form to discover the massive changes to the body's shape.

Through the Internet, I found Vanessa. I enjoyed listening to her thick Chilean accent, the roll of her *r*'s with a slight hoarseness to her voice. I guessed her to be in her thirties. She owned a company with her husband, located just outside Salt Lake City, where Karren lived. Perfect. Another reason to visit Karren.

I sent them detailed designs, precise measurements, and my mission statement. At first, as with Gabrielle, I felt the hesitation regarding the basic premise. They followed the usual M.O., starting with "What is she thinking?" followed by, "Oh, that's not a bad idea." Vanessa seemed to get a handle on what I wanted and was willing to work at a reasonable price. My team—Gabrielle and Vanessa—and I were in action.

Braiden and Chelsea's graduations were coming up, and coinciding with that, Gail's daughter was getting married, in Kentucky. This trip would be the perfect opportunity to debut my designs. For months we worked as a well-oiled machine, with Gabrielle and I alternating trips from her house to mine, and overnight Fed Ex packages traveling back and forth to Vanessa, filled with fabrics, drawings, and garments. I gave the complicated designs to Vanessa, and to Gabrielle, I gave the designs where getting the right fit on me was the important issue.

While we were working in my studio one day, Gabrielle clearly had something on her mind. She peered over her brightly colored reading glasses, which clashed with her just-dyed red hair and equally bright makeup.

"May I ask you to explain something?"

Oh boy, here it comes.

I was expecting, "Why would you not want breasts? Is that not the basis of our femininity?" I was formulating the answer in my mind. I would politely tell her that we could have our femininity without breasts. That this line of clothes would help us feel feminine.

"All of your designs use such drab colors, but your art is so colorful. Why is that?"

Not the question I was expecting.

She was right. My artwork surrounded us with color. The studio itself was vibrant, with the bright coral rug, the red hutch, and the deep red silk curtains framing the picture window. She would not understand that women like me did not want to stick out. We wanted to draw attention away from our bodies. The concept of the line was to confuse and blur the eye away from the chest area, not draw attention to it.

"My art and clothing are two different things. I'm blurring the body with my clothes. My art is an expression of joy." I was trembling inside. That was a plausible enough answer, I thought.

Gabrielle shrugged her shoulders, adjusted her glasses, and continued working.

Her question did get me thinking about the dichotomies in my life, as well as why I had spent so much time and energy changing my name, looking for a new persona. My name, my persona—both were something I could control. What I could not control was having no breasts.

Chapter Thirty-Two

Annie's Debut

*L*ife had presented the perfect opportunities to debut the line. First, I would attend Chelsea's graduation in the Twin Cities, then Braiden's graduation in DC, and finally, Gail's daughter's wedding in Kentucky.

Chelsea had a serious boyfriend, Andrew. I was impressed with anyone who could hold Chelsea's interest this long. His family would be at the graduation, and they would stay in Andrew's apartment, which was Andrew and Chelsea's excuse for Andrew staying with us. I had never slept in one of my daughter's apartments with a boyfriend, and it was tiny. *Tiny.* Not the best comfort zone for a crusader's debut.

Andrew's parents, grandparents, and newlywed sister and brother-in-law were coming, but I was the sole attendee from our family. The pressure was on. I had to be perfect. My clothes had to be perfect.

I was relieved that the weather was cool, and the tops stayed under a jacket. Even so, I was proud of what I had done.

"What do you do in Colorado?" was the question of the weekend.

"I'm designing a clothing line for breast cancer survivors." I felt comfortable leaving it at that, as they were busy with Andrew's graduation, and it looked like they were going to be part of Chelsea's life. Chelsea and Andrew were planning on moving to DC after graduation, and I did not want to scare them off with my fanatical rants about women and their breasts.

Braiden's graduation was next. She and Ben had recently moved in together. Both of my babies, shacking up!

When I arrived at their new home, she seemed happier and healthier than I had ever seen her. Her eyes glowed, and her tiny nose wrinkled as she smiled broadly.

"Close your eyes and hold out your hands," she said. Her entire body was wiggling, but with precision, she gently placed a long object in my outstretched hands.

She had given me one of the most valuable presents I have ever received—a handheld fan. It was a beautiful blue, an old-fashioned accordion fan that she had picked out at the National Gallery's gift shop (they have the best gift shop!). Perfect. I would be a sophisticated woman, fanning herself. It was May, in DC, which is notorious for its humidity and heat. This fan would keep me from passing out.

Luckily, it was unseasonably cool. The graduation ceremony went smoothly, and Braiden, Ben, and I enjoyed our time together.

During that visit, Braiden and I were shopping at Nordstrom when a saleswoman stopped us.

"That's a beautiful top."

"It's her design," Braiden put her arms on my shoulders and pushed me toward the woman.

"I design a line of clothes for breast cancer survivors, and this is one of the designs." My chest was huge, even without breasts. I was beaming.

"Oh my gosh," she continued, "my mother just had a mastectomy!"

Another sign!

I went into my spiel. She was intrigued.

"What do you charge for a top like that? Do you have a card?"

I had not gotten that far. *Think quickly.*

"It wholesales for about eighty dollars." Sounded good.

"Fair price," she noted. "I'll give this card to my mother. Thanks."

Nordstrom, the heart of fashion-conscious America, loving my clothes!

Not one to keep my triumphs to myself, I spent hours on the phone with every friend and relative. I had nothing to sell the woman or her mother, so I hoped that she would not call, but this was the validation I was looking for.

You would think I had won the Nobel Peace Prize. To me, I had.

Last stop on the agenda was Kentucky, an outdoor wedding—hot, humid, with a pending chance of tornados. And on the wedding day, we would be busy setting up. I imagined myself with ribbons of sweat pouring down my face (maybe people would mistake them for tears of happiness) and enormous round stains under my arms. But I somehow managed not to ruin the clothes during the setup.

My ensemble for the wedding was the epitome of everything I wanted to convey. A pleated chiffon top with strategically placed detailing took your eye away from the breasts and up toward the face. This was layered over a pleated camisole, mixing fabrics and pattern. A coordinating skirt took it to perfection. I danced the night away, confident that I had a great concept, great designs, and a great team. Annie Flats was here to give women the opportunity to "just be flat."

Soon I would be on to my next challenge. Chelsea and I were attending her childhood friend's wedding in Seattle. I wanted to push my designs harder, but sometimes I push too hard. Hence, the wallpaper dress was born.

Some of the choices I have made in clothing are especially embarrassing considering I am a clothing designer. I am either boring or way out there. This time I was way out there. The fabric was flowing and slightly sheer—and it called to me. A large geometric art deco print with shades of bluish purple and dull orange covered the fabric. It was pretty and would have looked grand on someone's wall, just not on my body.

But I loved it. I designed a simple short dress and put another dress over that. The underdress would peek out at the neck and the hem. It had pleats to give the illusion of breasts, while the wallpaper fabric skimmed over the body.

Here is the kicker. The underdress was chartreuse.

"Um. . . . . okay." Gabrielle winced. She expected weird designs from me, but this was over the top. Maybe so. I found a blue to match the pattern color, and Gabrielle made two underdresses, just to be on the safe side.

When she was finished, she cocked her head to one side, looking at the dresses. "The chartreuse actually looks good."

The wedding was a sea of tasteful neutrals. Even with the blue underdress, I stood out like a sore thumb, but I held my head high. Nothing I could do about it but hope our hosts would someday talk to me after I ruined their wedding photos. I never wore the wallpaper dress again, but I do get use out of the blue underdress. Not so much the chartreuse.

Chapter Thirty-Three

Annie Goes to Bloomingdale's

I could not shut up or stop working. I had verbal diarrhea of epic proportions with anyone who would or would not listen. Jamie was wearing out.

"Today I'm working on the fifth version of the third incarnation of the eighth design," I would report when I made my daily "Still alive" call.

"Mm hmm."

And when she managed to escape me, I'd call Karren, then Braiden. . . .

We were moving along, but I needed capital to make it a success. There are a zillion great designs and ideas, but the successful ones are backed up by investments. I decided to team up with a store that had production and advertising capabilities. They would line up for this opportunity, I thought. I envisioned racks of clothes, my logo in lights, and me on Oprah—again (because we'll have become best friends by then, of course).

I targeted a dozen stores that had the right image and

manufacturing capabilities, such as Bloomingdale's, Ann Taylor, and Liz Claiborne. I formulated a professional yet emotional letter and sent one to the top official in each company. My child was off to college—my idea was out in the world, on its own, ready for the taking.

After one week, three days, and eight and a half hours (but who's counting?), I received my first response—an email from the president of Bloomingdale's. Bloomingdale's! The president! He wanted me to meet with the vice president of fashion. The vice president of fashion!

I was on the phone again, calling friends, family, and probably some foes. Two days later I received an email from the vice president. I tried to convince myself that I would be happy just to get through the meetings without making a sweating, bumbling fool of myself, but I wanted a deal. I wanted a deal more than anything in the world. I would have sold my soul for a deal.

I was visiting the kids in DC and took a different bus to New York. I missed John (and my corned beef sandwich), but I didn't miss the drama.

It was the week of the presidential election. The air about DC and New York City was electric with anticipation. I stayed with Ty in Brooklyn my first night and woke up wanting the day to pass quickly. My meeting was the following day, and there was nothing more for me to do but wait.

"Let's watch *Gossip Girl*," Ty suggested. His voice and facial expressions were always just this side of exaggerated, giving the impression that he was really excited about whatever he was saying. But that was just Ty. Life was a stage.

"What's *Gossip Girl?*"

"It's a catty, gossipy show about rich, spoiled teenagers. You'll love it."

We spent the day lying on Ty's bed, watching episode after episode of one of the most mindless shows I have ever seen. It was perfect.

I rehearsed my spiel over and over again and practiced breathing exercises to stay calm and dry. That evening, Ty drove me to the northern end of Manhattan, where I would spend the night and the remainder of the trip with my college roommate from Parsons, the New York design school I'd attended until I moved out to San Diego. She and her husband seemed as excited as I was about the meeting. They were the perfect people to be with.

The next morning, they drove me up to the front door of Bloomingdale's. I was ready. I wore one of my tops, sleek black pants, and a slick leather blazer. My samples were in a black garment bag, and I carried a simple black leather purse and black leather portfolio. My hands were full, but I was determined to pull this meeting off with style and grace. I was a boobless old fashionista.

I was twenty minutes early, so I decided to walk around the sales floor to soak up the atmosphere—and soak up any sweat. I sauntered across the sales floor, with the clear knowledge that this was where my clothing and I belonged. As I was relishing my place in this world, my portfolio slipped out of my arms, plummeted to the ground, and scattered across the floor. Drawings everywhere. *Stay calm.* I picked up the pages, one by one. With as much grace as I could muster, I carried my precious cargo against my chest to a corner of the store and put the portfolio back together. I was not sweating. *Breathe.*

I found the office, where the vice president greeted me politely and showed me into a meeting room. She was older than I thought she would be but looked every bit the part of the New York classic fashionista. In many department store offices, the employees are very young; a buyer can be in her early twenties, so I hadn't known whether I would find a trendy young upstart or a clone from the book *The Devil Wears Prada.* She was neither.

Relieved, I hung up my samples and gave her a copy of my mission statement. I was surprised when she took the time to read it. I removed my blazer to be proactive about the sweat factor, and when she was ready, I spoke slowly and calmly, explaining my concept and each design. The presentation was flawless. She listened intently while taking notes. Notes are a good sign.

She gave thought to what she was about to say.

"What are your production costs?"

My excitement intensified.

"I want to work with an organization that already has production capabilities, so we can keep the production costs down," I answered, hoping that she would volunteer to make Bloomingdale's my vehicle for success.

"We don't manufacture anything."

Okay. . . . we can overcome this. Just give me the orders, and I will find a way.

"Your line is beautiful," she continued. "The concept and idea that you have is commendable, but I don't feel that it's suited for a large store such as ours. It's a very personal product, which needs to be explained by a trained salesperson on a one-to-one, personal level, someone who can take the time to explain the product and concept. I think it would do better in a small boutique."

The meeting lasted an hour and a half, during which I spoke clearly and eloquently, without breaking a sweat. I had not sold the line or the concept, but I had conquered the sweat. Her comments made sense, and I would process them and move forward.

Her favorite design? The wallpaper dress.

The remainder of the visit was just for fun. I spent more time with Ty and friends. I was swept up in the joy of the city when it was announced that Obama had won the election. Our new president and I were on our way to saving the world.

I heard from the other stores and manufacturers. No interest, but I was not discouraged; all I needed was one break, and it was just a matter of time and perseverance. I had lots of the latter. In high school, I had been a loner, and when it was time to sign yearbooks, I was desperate for someone to sign mine. I asked my art teacher, whom I idolized, to sign it. He did not seem very excited about it, but I ignored his hesitation. He scribbled, "To Lynne, who refuses to be ignored."

Chapter Thirty-Four

Standing Naked in Front of Class

I was not getting the joint ventures I hoped for. My twelve complex designs needed to go down to six less-costly designs, a more manageable size for funding.

Ideas flowed, from developing a website, to wholesale sales, to specialty stores, to home party distribution, or a combination. Every day I got on the bandwagon of a different way to market, hoping that at some point, the path would organically appear. As a Chanukah present, Ben and Jamie surprised me with a website for Annie Flats. I could send an email with a link to the website to all my contacts and to anyone who would give me their email address. It would just be a matter of time before the word would get out, and mastectomy survivors everywhere would see the beauty of going flat. It was a grass-roots approach; I had a global solution in mind, but I would take it. It was a step.

I was up and down, one day committed to the website, and another, coming up with money that I did not have to attend a health industry trade show in North Carolina. The trade show route would mean selling to small specialty stores, and I would need a manufacturer who could handle small quantities. Vanessa had a connection with a small manufacturer. Mind you, two hundred pieces was the minimum quantity, which was too many pieces for me to manufacture on my own, but if I had orders, it could work. It was a risk, but if I wanted to succeed, I had to take the chance.

The trade show in North Carolina would be expensive, especially with airfare, but I decided to do it. I designed a booth that would be inexpensive and easy to transport. I purchased inexpensive dress forms to perform mastectomies on. It was going to be a lot of work to perform three, but I was a top-notch surgeon. The forms would show how my designs worked.

I gave Gabrielle and Vanessa new designs to work on. The old designs were good, but I needed ones suitable for manufacturing in small quantities. While Vanessa and Gabrielle worked on the garments, and I waited for my surgery patients to arrive, I designed a new logo and hangtag.

A month before the show, I went to visit my mother in San Diego. Karren joined us. Then she and I would fly to Salt Lake together, where I would meet Vanessa to work together in person. I wanted Karren at the meeting, even though I was uncomfortable with my fat ill-shaped body next to hers. I valued her opinion. I was also nervous about exposing my body to Vanessa. She had my measurements, so she knew what my body looked like, but only on paper. I kept reminding myself that to succeed, I would have to sacrifice my modesty.

I ordered a sizable quantity of bamboo fabric, thinking ahead to manufacturing, but when I opened the box, wrong color—cream. Panic. I checked the order slip—black. Clearly, this was not black. How could they get *that* wrong? Vanessa needed the fabric ASAP, and it was Friday afternoon, so the fabric offices were closed. I would have to wait until Monday morning.

Early Monday, a new shipment was on its way. It was the right color, but this time the fabric had holes in it. They had sent additional yardage to compensate, but the holes where in random places, making the fabric impossible to use for manufacturing. I sent it to Vanessa. She could make the samples, and there would be time after I took the orders to correct the problem. These things happen.

Although I wanted to believe that the designs were good, in the back of my mind, I knew better, but I ignored these thoughts and moved forward. It was D-day: I was about to show the garments that Gabrielle had made to Karren and my mother. The designs were far from perfect, but they could be refined later. The fabric, even though it was my wonder fabric, had somehow lost life when it became a garment. The clothes were soft, antibacterial, and made of sustainable fabric to boot, but they were drab—even for me—and lifeless. I didn't want to go out there, but my mother and Karren were waiting.

It was like those nightmares when you are standing naked in front of a class. Only this was real.

I stood in front of the kitchen table. My mother and Karren forced a smile.

Silence, except for the sound of Mom scraping the bottom of her bowl of fruit with her spoon.

"Well, it's a start." Karren adjusted her taupe glasses, her clear blue eyes still a striking feature behind them. Her hair was now a solid white, short and spiky. "I'm not sure it's exactly what you want."

"It's not your best look," my mother chimed in. She refused to give in to wearing glasses and had deep wrinkles between her eyes from always squinting. Her gray shoulder length hair was pulled back and fastened with an exotic clip she had found at a garage sale.

"Let's analyze this." Karren pursed her lips in thought. "It has some good ideas, but I think you need to keep working on it."

She always insisted that I push myself beyond my first try and learn from my trials, not expecting every effort to be a winner. It drove me nuts, but unfortunately, this time she was right.

My mother was out of her chair, tucking, pulling, and gathering the garment. She was in her late eighties but had the agility of a thirty-year-old.

Then I felt hot flashes taking over. I wanted to rip the clothes off and throw myself into baggy sweats, never to come out of them again.

We all knew. It was not coming together. All I heard was chatter, and all I wanted to do was cry.

Karren's eyes softened. "Maybe you should think about not going to the show."

There it was.

"Maybe you should pull out and not rush it. It would be better to lose the deposit than to spend a tremendous amount of money and time to show up with a product you won't be proud of."

She was right. I phoned my rock, Jamie, who agreed. "I'm sorry, but they're right. I didn't want to say anything, but they're right. The designs just aren't that great. It would be best to pull out of the show, work hard until they're perfect, and go to the show next year."

It was heart wrenching, but I canceled. Deep down I had known long before this day, but I needed my support group to give me a dose of reality. I could not do it myself.

I was still scheduled to visit Vanessa to fit her garments, and it made sense to continue, but I openly doubted myself. The basic premise of the line was in question. It was not just that the fit was wrong. The fit was wrong because maybe, just maybe, a woman needs breasts to get the right proportions. Was it possible that I needed breasts? My clothes looked like gobs of fabric across my chest. The shape does not undulate in and out, like breasts do. The design does not flow around my body, blending into the side and back.

I had a front and a back, but no depth. I was two-dimensional but needed to be three.

What was happening? Was I a traitor to my own cause?

No. I had to move on.

Vanessa's studio was in a modern office building near Salt Lake City. I had guessed right about her being in her thirties. She was dressed in a classic but funky style, much hipper than I would have thought of someone living in a small Utah town. This was conservative country, the home of Brigham Young and the Mormon Church. She and her husband had come to the States from Chile, probably through the church. Karren noticed the traditional Mormon underclothes beneath

Vanessa's funky outfit. What a dichotomy.

Vanessa and I went into a side office so that I could change into the first top. She seemed excited to see her creations on this strange person.

Here I was, old, not the trimmest person in the world, deformed, about to undress in front of one of the cutest, most fashionable women I had met in a long time. I had a tank top on under my shirt, but she would clearly see that I was misshapen and flat.

Suck it up. It was going to be worth it. I needed to do this so my disciples could proclaim their breastless freedom.

She seemed uninterested in my damaged body. The new garments were tight, and getting in and out of them required her help. I began to sweat from embarrassment, tussling with the clothing, and hot flashes. One thing I can count on is for hot flashes to come at the most inopportune times, and my flashes, also known as power surges, were a work of art. First the sweat—lots of it. So much for my pristinely placed makeup. Then came the red. Not just a flush, but big, bright, Rudolph-the-red-nosed-reindeer red. And not a full-face flush (I can't believe that I would wish for a uniform flush). Imagine your cheek with a neon red perfect square. Just your cheek. As though you'd applied your entire case of blush in a deliberate square with perfect ninety-degree angles.

I was a sweaty, neon, flat potato trying to squeeze into a tight sack.

Karren, Vanessa's husband, and their assistant sat in chairs placed along the long wall of a rectangular waiting room. I came out and stood at one end.

I was standing in front of everyone, including the spirit of Monica Silverman, whose body Karren's reminded me of. I had a choice at that moment—skulk away or embrace the situation and get over it. It was time to get over it. Monica Silverman was no longer going to control my self-image. My body was not so bad for a fifty-eighty-year-old. I still had a waist, and a flat stomach. What more could anyone ask for?

Monica Silverman had nothing on me.

Vanessa's husband took notes as I played fit model and we made corrections to the garment. Karren looked on and added her opinions.

"Is it tight here and loose there?" Vanessa and her assistant pulled and tugged. Straight pins held between their lips flew with lightning speed to nip and tuck where needed. Vanessa's thick wavy hair flipped frantically from side to side.

"I think the pattern needs to scoop more here." I pointed to places that needed work. We had completely different backgrounds and lives, yet we had fashion and patternmaking in common, and for this moment, we spoke the same language. Comrades.

Yet, I was unhappy with the garments. Or was it the premise?

Karren and I drove to her house along the gorgeous Front Range Mountains of Utah

"Where should we eat tonight?"

"I don't know. How about Rio Grande or Barbacoa?"

"Who has the best margarita?"

"Rio Grande."

"Rio Grande it is."

191

World peace–level problem solved.

Our conversation then ventured back to the clothing line, and that led to body image.

"I've never told anyone," Karren confided. "But as a kid, I never took dance classes because I didn't think my body was feminine enough."

Doesn't every girl want to dance? She had never allowed herself because she did not feel feminine. Wow. She was beautiful. Her body was perfect. I never loved my body, but that never stopped me. I was damaged, but I felt feminine. Go figure.

In the end, this trip had made me feel better about my body, better than I'd felt in decades. But I was not feeling better about Annie Flats. There were cracks in my crusade.

Chapter Thirty-Five

A Perfect Tee

I was carrying boxes of fabric up the tight stairs from the basement. My "now not so wonder" fabric had traveled up and down many times now, from studio to storage, storage to studio. It was getting used to the routine.

"Going to try again?" Jamie called out wearily as she came in through the kitchen door. She was getting sick of the routine. Even Rowena seemed bored.

The clothing line had gotten smaller, down to three pieces at best, and even those I was not happy with. I tried to develop new styles, even sewed them myself. I could not justify putting any more money into this.

"How long did it take you this time?" She groaned as she turned the corner, grabbing a box that had been positioned precariously on top of another box, just about ready to tumble back down the stairs.

"Three days," I muttered. "I'm getting better. I only lasted a day the last time."

"You and that damn line."

All our frustration levels were mounting. I would not let myself consider that to get the look of breasts, you need breasts. I would box everything up, put away the hateful sewing machine, cart it all downstairs to the basement, and walk away. This was the way I handled frustration. Packing things away. Moving furniture. But it never lasted very long. I would lug it all back up to my studio to try again. My mission had become an unhealthy obsession, but I was getting good exercise.

I stayed up late and got up early. Sleep was not in my vocabulary. Neither was cleaning, showering, or socializing. Jamie and my walks with Carolyn and Linda were my only outside life. I piled the failed samples on top of each other to make my sewing chair more comfortable. With each discarded garment, Mona became happier and happier with her ever-rising bed. I went from cardigans to jackets to T-shirts. I thought, talked, and did nothing else.

Jamie was ready to disown me. I tried, not very successfully, to temper my clothing talk. Her life revolved around her new obsession, a ginormous breed of dog called Tibetan mastiffs. Let me tell you, these dogs are huge. And just as independent as her yaks. She loved a challenge. So I made an effort to talk about them to earn points to allow me to talk about my clothes.

My "still alive" calls to Jamie got shorter and shorter.

"Which dog escaped today?"

"Today it was Spudgy, but yesterday, Keniky jumped out my car window. With the window almost completely closed."

"Uh huh. I think I need to make the pleats smaller on the latest top. Got to run, bye."

Linda and Carolyn were captive audiences on our walks.

"I started a new painting yesterday."

"Are you doing horses again?"

"I didn't get that far. I got as far as painting the background, then the canvas ended up in a corner to make room for the sewing machine."

"I thought you put the sewing machine away"

"I did. But it came upstairs. It missed me."

"So what design are you working on?'

"A version of the cardigan that I worked on a few weeks ago."

"A cardigan would be good. They can be worn year-round."

"Yeah, you're right. Let's stop at the coffee shop. They might have a leftover bagel for Tula."

My life was a routine of fitful nights, walking, working on the patterns, sewing, cussing at the sewing machine, boxing up the fabrics and sewing machine, bringing the boxes downstairs, walking, bringing the boxes upstairs, cussing at the sewing machine, walking, cussing, bringing the boxes downstairs, and finally, at the end of that day, brooding through the long night.

Then the light went on. I would narrow my scope even more and design the holy grail of clothing—the perfect tee. Every woman loves a T-shirt of some sort, and mine would be the perfect tee for women like me. As I carried the boxes of fabric, the sewing machine, and my tools upstairs, it came to me. A T-shirt would be an ideal giveaway item for Bloomingdale's cancer awareness promotion. Bloomingdale's had not seen the last of me. Once I had the slightest door opening, I was going to sink my teeth into it with the grip of a bulldog. My crusade would be saved. I was pumped up. I worked feverishly to design my perfect tee. I tore apart shirts that had a good fit to copy their pattern and draped neckline after neckline, working to create a garment worthy of Bloomingdale's.

I was planning to spend the summer in DC and was determined to send a sample to Bloomingdale's before I left. Imperfect tees were strewn everywhere. I even eliminated walks as I narrowed in on my conquest.

The final design was exquisitely simple. A large cowl neck cascaded down the chest to hide the flat body beneath. The neckline had the perfect amount of fabric and drape. The bodice was form fitting but not tight. It curved in at the waist and tapered gently out, stopping just above the hips. The sleeves were three-quarter length and hit the arm at the most flattering point. I had just enough of my bamboo fabric to make the final one, and it was perfect.

I revised the hangtag and logo yet again and composed an irresistible letter to Bloomingdale's. Everything was perfect; even my sewing was acceptable. I coddled my baby in pink tissue with a pink bow to symbolize the breast cancer fight.

Then, with a deep breath, I handed the package to the Fed Ex man.

Chapter Thirty-Six

The Real Reveal

*B*loomingdale's response came quickly.

Not interested.

Undeterred, I prepared for a summer in DC. At nineteen, when I had left DC to go to college in New York City, I had sworn I would never move back. But, much to my surprise, I loved the city, plus both girls and their boyfriends lived there. We had been spread out all over the world, and now we could be together. Braiden was taking the summer off from working on her PhD, and these would be Chelsea's last free months before starting her career. It made sense to go now, but the thought of moving to DC was daunting, especially considering the hot, humid summers. I was spending the summer there to see how I would handle it.

My perfect tee would get me through.

Once again, I had too many cars. Chelsea had used our Camry while in law school, but after she graduated, it came back to me. I had the SUV that I had purchased in Montana, and the old SUV had 267,000 miles on it and was in semi-retirement. I decided to drive the Camry to DC for Braiden to use for commuting to school. She flew out to Colorado to keep me company on the long drive. Tula would come with us, and my nephew and his girlfriend would stay at my house to keep Mona company.

"Road trip!"

Alan and I had raised our family on road trips to our favorite mountains and lakes, but this time we were headed east, through uncharted territory. Braiden and I were excited about the new terrain as well as about spending time together.

We sang at the top of our lungs to "I Love You Always Forever" and Ricky Martin, and we held our breath as we drove through treacherous thunderstorms. We stopped at the arch in St. Louis, and I ran up the stairs like Rocky, with Tula at my side. Da da daaaaaaaaa, da da daaaaa. It was "umpossible" to think that I would fail in my mission.

Upon arrival, we went to register the Camry, since DC loved to tow away out-of-state cars. The DMV was in Georgetown, which in the sixties had been a conclave of hippy boutiques but was now full of high end chain stores.

"I have to get my driver's license plus register the car, so this will take a while," Braiden said, rummaging through her purse. "I think I have all the documents I'll need. It's amazing what I can fit in here." At any one time, she had an assortment of bags, purses, and scarves slung across her thin shoulders.

"The mall has some stores you might like," she said. "Maybe you'll find something for the summer."

"Great idea." I actually liked the chain stores better than the boutiques. There was more anonymity, and I did not feel so guilty when I inevitably returned the item. "Call me when you're done."

I sauntered off to play sophisticated city woman. I was the epitome of style with my meticulously applied makeup and my perfect tee. I was a fashionable "mature" woman who fit flawlessly into upscale Georgetown.

The mall had been added to the Georgetown landscape to look like a street scene out of the 1800s. Ornate patinaed grillwork and greenery lined the brick walkways, which opened onto a three-level covered courtyard. Old-fashioned lampposts added light, although it paled in comparison to the rays of sunlight coming through the skylights.

I arched my chest, my beautifully disguised body displayed for all.

Then it happened.

It happened so fast.

I caught my reflection in a window. *Who was that person?*

I continued on to another window that had paper covering the inside, thinking I could get a better look.

I was horrified.

The draped collar made me look like a clown. A misshapen, flat, freakish clown. My fabric had betrayed me and was clinging to the undulating scar tissue, and my chest looked like a lumpy, stuffed sack of potatoes. The collar accentuated the wide expanse of my breastless chest beneath a sagging sweaty face that had lost all remnants of the makeup I had meticulously applied.

I was mortified and embarrassed, but even worse than that was what I was thinking.

I want breasts.

I. Want. Breasts.

I wanted to abandon all my not-yet-found disciples. I wanted to go under the knife and put foreign objects into my body. I wanted to give up what I had felt to the bottom of my heart was my mission in life. I wanted to abandon all of womankind. How could I even consider this? It was a betrayal of monumental proportion.

Maybe I was dehydrated. I was hallucinating. If I kept walking, the reflection would change. After all, walking had always been my savior. The heat emanating from my face was unbearable. The sweat seared across it, the fabric clung, and there was nothing I could do but hope that some window would transform me back to the woman I thought I was.

And what was I thinking? I want breasts?

I could not fully admit this blasphemy to myself, let alone to anyone else. I could not stand living with my body, and I could not stand to think what I was thinking. Days went by as I grappled with my thoughts.

Finally, I came clean.

"Lynne," Jamie said gently, "You've given this your all. You needed to go through this process and figure out what you wanted. You needed to be your obsessed self and come out wherever that took you. Unfortunately, you've realized what you didn't want to hear. You have a noble cause with no market. Not even yourself."

She was right.

Chapter Thirty-Seven

Aw, It's Your First Bra . . . Again

*B*raiden was next on my confessional list. We sat in their tiny IKEA chairs in the living room. It amazed me that Braiden, five-foot seven, and Ben, six-foot eight (not a typo), could contort themselves, with much grace I might add, to each fit perfectly into a chair with the little chair arm curled around them. The arms were embracing me now.

"I want breasts. Just like all the other women." I still could not believe what I was saying.

"When I see myself in the mirror, I see a deformed potato." I teared up.

"Mom." Ever so gently, she moved her chair closer to mine. "I was only ten when you had your first mastectomy. And it was only two years later when you had your second, so I don't remember you with breasts." Her body was uncharacteristically still. No wiggling or tapping. "After your mastectomy and all the trouble it caused you, I could see your discomfort with yourself. We would all be at a party, and I would notice you."

I looked up for a second, my eyes widening, then looked down in embarrassment.

She leaned forward to tuck a stray lock of my hair out of my red face. "Although to the outside world you looked confident, I could see this . . . awkwardness that told me you were not happy with your body." She put her hand on mine and squeezed. "It's okay that you want to be like everyone else," she said. "It's okay. You're a wonderful, beautiful person. It doesn't matter if you have breasts or not. Whatever you want. What we do want is for you to be happy and healthy. That's all that matters."

This is my beautiful child, I thought. *I'm so damn lucky.*

We reached across the arms of the chairs and gave each other a hug. Tears welled up in my eyes, and she used the sleeve of her blouse to wipe away a stray drop on my cheek. Our eyes met, then we both looked down at our bodies, awkwardly stretched across the once-white arms of the chairs, and burst into laughter.

"We need ice cream," I said. I wanted to crawl into a hole and eat fatty, sugary foods. And move furniture. I wanted to be depressed. I wanted to wallow in self-pity.

But that was not what I was going to do. I would return to the land of the bras. And I needed to do it *now*.

Braiden took me to Saks to see her bra fitter, Ellen. Just another mother (Braiden) taking her preteen daughter (that would be me) to her favorite bra fitter for that special first bra. Ellen had fit both girls and could tell which size and style fit best with just a glance. I reasoned that if anyone could figure out how to fit me, she could.

It did not hurt that she was a bit older than me; I did not have to confront the cute little hard-body salesgirl usually found at department stores or the overly compassionate saleswomen at prosthesis stores, where I felt damaged, surrounded by reminders of cancer. I was not going to go back to that. I was going to move forward. I wanted to be like every other breasted woman and go to the lingerie department of a nice store.

DC's Saks was located in an area known for its upscale shopping, housing such stores as Tiffany, Gucci, and Cartier. Once understatedly elegant, now the area was more about status. Beautiful young ladies, dressed to kill and shop, mixed with the aging intellectuals of the political elite.

The lingerie department, located on the basement floor of Saks, looked like any other department store lingerie area—except that it housed Ellen. She was helping another woman and politely acknowledged us as we entered her department. The customer seemed to be in her fifties, heavily made up and wearing a flowing sheer silk blouse neatly tucked into her skinny white jeans, which accentuated her size 00 body. She was dressed to impress, and she looked as though she had cosmetic surgery bills to match. As she sized me up, taking in my frumpy clothes, she probably wondered what these peons were doing in *her* store and why they were standing near her. In actuality, she probably was not thinking of me at all, but at the time, I felt as though the entire world was focused on me and that fact that I was about to get boobs.

Braiden and I wandered off to look around while we waited. Ellen's customer was going to take as long as she could. Make the lowly common folk wait.

Finally, Ellen approached us with a warm grin on her face, her graying hair neatly tied back.

"I've had a double mastectomy, and I need new breasts," I blurted. Just get it out there. Red was chomping at the bit to take control of my face. Sweat was not far behind.

Ellen gave Braiden a compassionate glance.

"What size cup would you like?" she asked, unfazed, in her New York accent. It was a familiar accent that gave me a scant bit of comfort in this excruciatingly uncomfortable situation.

What size would I like off the menu? Something from column A or column B?

With as much pride as I could muster, and trying not to shake too much, I said, "I used to be an A or a B cup, so I guess that's what I'll be."

"That sounds like a place to start." Ellen held her slim arm out and motioned for us to go into the dressing room while she went on the search for bras.

"Let's start with these," she said as she knocked on the dressing room door. She brought four different styles. "These are all the same size but fit differently." Even though Ellen looked discreetly toward the floor, I kept my tank top on until she left. I was not ready to show Ellen my scars.

Moment of truth. I had not worn a bra, nonetheless tried one on at Saks, for almost twenty years. Braiden's deliberately looked around the room as I removed my tank and tried on my first challenge, a lacy number.

What wonders a bit of lace can do. I was feeling a bit sassy. *Look at me, I am a sexy WOMAN!*

But the cups were big and empty. Braiden's ponytail brushed across her shoulder as she turned to see how it looked.

Silence.

"There's something missing here." I poked at the collapsing cups of the bra.

"No kidding." Braiden rolled her eyes. "Guess you'll have to get boobs."

Guess so.

I could fill those holes. I had acquired expertise at creating breasts while lopsided. My favorite material for breasts in the olden days, shoulder pads, were out of fashion. Rolled-up pantyhose might do, but I wanted real fake boobs, not improvised boobs. I was not going to mess around with this. It was real fake boobs or nothing at all.

I had a plan in place. I had researched online what was available in prostheses. I was not willing to wait for an online order, and there was a specialty bra and prosthesis store near Saks. I would pick up some cheap boobs there. But my bra would not come from a prosthesis store. *No.* I was going to get my bra from Saks.

I tried on a different style, with pointy tips. The size was the same, but Oh My God. I felt like I had double Ds.

"I've got torpedoes!"

"Wow, Mom, you're stacked."

I continued to wrestle with each new bra-venture while Braiden fidgeted with her shoe strap, dumpster dove in her bottomless purse, and braided her hair in three different ways. It was strange how the potential breasts inhibited movement. Every time I moved my arms, there were breasts in the way. It was like a stack of books was protruding from my chest and my arms could not get around it.

There we stood, Ellen and Braiden watching as I swung my arms from side to side, all the while brushing up against the pointy cones jutting out from my chest. Ellen's delicate head tilted to one side as she stood by the door opening, as if to say, "There's no way I'm entering the room with this crazy lady." I could hear Braiden's peeps as she tried to hold in her squeaks of laughter. When she could not hold it in anymore, shrill gasps for air penetrated the dressing room area. A fifty-eight-year-old mother of two was rediscovering the world of breasts with all the naiveté of a preteen.

I tried on a few more bras, narrowing it down to two. One was demure, with lace trim. It gave me little bumps of breasts. The other one looked hot, a bit too hot for the first time out. I was not ready for that. I picked the baby bumps.

"It's the new you. And you need to wear the bra now." Braiden was already out the dressing room door. I followed dutifully.

"Mom, come this way, you're headed for the kid's section." She put her hands gently on my shoulders to guide me in the right direction. "You're white as a ghost."

The entire store must have known that this old lady had just bought her first bra. How stupid and pathetic is she? I tried to hold my head high, tried to keep calm and not walk into anyone or anything with my newly launched torpedoes.

I was exhausted, but I caught my breath, and we headed to the specialty store to purchase my new breasts. It was a small, cramped store, filled with bathing suits and no mention of us "special women." I was thankful for the discretion but not excited to see rows of bikinis and young women with perfect bodies milling about. The only salesperson was a twenty-something, thin, blonde girl who behaved as though this were her first job. Clearly she had no idea what she was doing, and clearly she was not the one I wanted to deal with. It seemed like forever before she acknowledged us, and when I explained that all I wanted were the inexpensive prostheses I had seen on their website, she looked at me with a dazed "deer in the headlights" stare. Nothing between those pretty little ears.

"The owner of the store will have to fit you," she said, emotionless, "and she's out to lunch, and I don't know what time she gets back."

Great. I wanted to get it over with, so all we could do was wait. Wait, wait, wait. We watched young girls buy bikinis. We watched old ladies buy one-piece bathing suits.

Finally the owner appeared. She must have weighed eighty pounds soaking wet. She was definitely going for the "I'll do whatever I have to do to stay young looking" look. Tons of makeup, many hours in the gym, and probably many hours at the plastic surgeon. Just what I needed. She went to help someone else, not in any hurry to help us. Braiden kept her cool, but I was just about at the end of my rope. I wanted to buy my damn boobs and go.

When it was our turn to be honored by the owner's presence, I gave her my usual spiel. This woman had no sense of humor, no emotion, and no interest other than to sell. She had a set routine, and veering from it was not an option.

"We don't know what size you'll need until you try them on," she said coldly. "Plus, you need a special bra. We have those."

It did not matter that I had my Saks bag in my hand, a small bag, just the size of a bra. It also did not matter that I said I had a bra and did not need the special bras with the pockets for the new breasts. And it certainly did not help when she said, "Oh, by the way, we carry the brand of bra that you just bought from Saks."

I just wanted my boobs, please.

"Mom, please, try their bra on. Please, just do it." The dark circles under her eyes were starting to show. She was tired, I was tired and emotionally worn out, and I wanted to go home.

Fine. Give me your damn bra.

I was handed a medium-size prosthesis and a bra that looked like the torturous Playtex Living bras for well-endowed women. If there was one thing I was not, it was well endowed. The bra was an armored tank, but I was determined to get through this and tried it on, along with the medium breasts. Wow, was I big! I mean huge! They really got in the way. I could not imagine myself accomplishing anything in my life with these enormous mountains.

And then I heard Braiden's squeal, once again trying to hide her laughter. We would be okay.

I politely asked for the smaller size breast. Reluctantly, the owner brought it. They were not much bigger than the shoulder pads I used to use, and they were twice as expensive, but I needed them now. I needed to experience breasts *now*. A day, a week, a month from now was not acceptable. And I could not wear one of those special bras. I needed a beautiful, feminine bra.

Oh, and by the way, after doing a little research, I have discovered that the best price for fake boobs is at Walgreens. com. You got it, Walgreens, the drug store, has prostheses online. Who would have thought?

Chapter Thirty-Eight

Do You Think I Need to Wear Boobs with This Dress?

My new breasts were mosquito bites, but they felt like mountains. Every time I moved my arms, my "huge" chest got in the way. My daughters watched me with puzzlement as I clumsily maneuvered my way around my breasts.

I realized that I had to face the boyfriends, who knew I was flat. My brain told me that they really could not care less about my vacillating positions on breasts. I was an old lady, their girlfriend's mother, so staring at my chest was the last thing on their minds. But I was embarrassed. All they had heard from me since we met was how committed I was to this cause. Now all of sudden, poof! I was done with that?

How would I face them with torpedoes suddenly in their faces? Would I proclaim my new body parts and get the awkwardness over in one fell swoop? Or go about my business, not saying a word, yet knowing that my daughters have told their boyfriends that Mom has boobs.

I was familiar with awkward stares from men and women and chuckled when it was clear that someone was trying not to look at my breasts. They would look into my eyes only to have human nature bully their eye muscles into looking down.

My first outing with my breasts was under a baggy shirt. With trepidation and the Himalayas on my chest, I marched down the stairs.

Ben was sitting at the dining room table, working on his computer.

"I have breasts."

"That's nice; you look great," he said nonchalantly.

His perfectly styled dark hair did not move an inch as he lifted his head, eyes still focused on his computer. There was not the slightest notion of interest in my new breasts.

The glow from my fluorescent cheeks must have been brighter than his computer screen. Shaking, I took a deep breath. I felt embarrassed about my narcissistic moment and headed back up the stairs.

Then it was Andrew's turn. I had already come clean to Chelsea.

"Mom, we love you no matter what your body looks like." The red curls she'd had as a child had been straightened and cut into a sophisticated, chin-length auburn bob. She did not talk much, but when she did, it was powerful.

"You know that whatever you decide, we will back you and love you,"

There was always comfort in hugging Chelsea. Her solid body just knew how to hug.

Chelsea and Andrew had invited us over for dinner. Fortunately, I was bringing Tula, whom they both loved, so the attention was on her as I marched nervously into the apartment.

"I have breasts."

"Uh huh."

It was now on to the real world, beyond the safety of lingerie departments and family. Birdie was in town and had invited me to the theater, which would be a proper first outing for my new breasts. I chose a loose fitting blouse that I was comfortable wearing without boobs and carefully positioned the bra and prostheses into place.

As I awkwardly maneuvered into the passenger seat, I was concerned that the bra or the prostheses would move around. Just what I needed on my first night out—my bra twisting sideways, or the enormous (in my mind only) prosthetic boobs popping out, with me unable to catch them. But I managed to get in the car and buckled up without incident.

We had barely moved twenty-five feet before I proclaimed, yet again:

"Look, I have boobs!"

She was driving through city traffic, so she kept her eyes on the road, even though I could see I had taken her by surprise. She could always keep her cool, so I wasn't sure if she was processing what I had said or if she was just paying attention to traffic. After a moment or so, she answered, her tone an odd mix of proud and confused:

"So do I."

Maybe this would not be so hard after all.

I spent most of the summer experimenting with wearing a bra and not wearing one.

"Do you think I need to wear boobs with this dress?"

Braiden would roll her eyes. "Yes, Mom. No, Mom. Either way, Mom." Not a day went by when that question was not asked.

At first the prostheses stayed on the shelf. I was too self-conscious about my torpedoes. I felt like they said, look at me! Fake breasts! I was also worried that they would pop out of my shirt if I moved too quickly or twisted in the wrong way, or that they'd slowly creep up my bra to peek out of my shirt.

I wished I still had implants. But at least my fake boobs would not deflate. I wondered how many women had flats. When I had my implant, I would think about what type of impact it would take to deflate the pouch. It had been under my muscle tissue, which definitely protected it, but after all, they were just plastic bags with saline water in them, so something could conceivably pop them, like in the episode of *Will and Grace* when Grace wore a water-enhanced bra to make her look larger and the water bags burst. There I would be, just like her, with water spouting from my breast. But it didn't matter. Implants were not an option for me. My body had stated loud and clear that they were unacceptable.

For years I had been as flat as a board, and that was where I was comfortable. I went on a few first dates from the Internet, and each time, I chose not to wear a bra. I think I just wanted to be comfortable in a stressful environment, but maybe it was a litmus test. A man who liked me flat chested was a man who wanted to get to know me, not my body. Come on now, really,

Lynne. At sixty and seventy, single men probably just want a woman who is breathing. Breasts are probably not the first, or even the last, things on their minds. Anyway, by my age even the best breasts were headed south and not very pretty.

The tops I wore when flat chested looked terrible with breasts. I still wanted to hide under my baggy shirts, but as my confidence increased, the clothes became more fitted. Living in the city helped. In Colorado I could get away with wearing the baggiest shirt I could find. I spent my life in a messy art studio, at the grocery store, walking, or on my sister's ranch. Who cared what I wore? Not the yaks.

But I do like the way I feel when dressed in clothes that make me look as good as I can. I feel better about myself, and I think I project that. As unfair as it is, people treat you differently depending on how you are dressed. I am also continuing to realize that this body is not so bad, especially for my age. My waist is smallish, my tummy is flat, and now with my new body addition, my waist is shapelier, my tummy looks flatter.

Karren used to give me a hard time for always changing the cabinet pulls in the houses I lived in. I could practically hear the roll of her eyes over the phone as she sarcastically agreed that yes, tiny little cabinet pulls made a drastic difference in a huge room. In my mind they did, and in my mind, these tiny little bags of polyester fiberfill made a huge difference on me. It's all in the details.

My body is no longer two-dimensional. No longer just large and wide. No longer just up and down. Now it is three-dimensional. Up, down, and out. It is amazing to me. Even my mosquito bites make a difference.

Chapter Thirty-Nine

Mom, You're Migrating

*M*y minimal summer wardrobe left much to be desired, especially now that my perfect tee was in the trash and I had breasts.

Braiden and I went to Loehmann's, a discount store where you could find designer clothes at discount prices. I had my bra from Saks, and I had added a comfortable sports bra, but I wanted more bras. More bras meant more normalcy.

We waited in line for a private dressing room, but the wait was long, it was hot, and I was dreading trying on bras. I began eyeing Loehmann's communal dressing room, which filled me with an entirely different kind of dread.

Braiden looked at me compassionately. "We'll do whatever you want," she said softly.

"Let's just do it," I said. "I'm hot and tired. Let's get it over with."

It was midday on a Thursday, so I was hoping the room would be empty, but there was a twenty-something girl in there, trying on dresses. She was of average height and not stocky but far from thin. She obviously worked hard to achieve her look, with lots of makeup and brown- and blonde-streaked hair teased into a mass of waves.

The thought of exposing myself in front of anyone, much less this young lady, who clearly cared about appearance, was daunting. I hesitated. Finally I decided there was no room for modesty after giving birth to two children and having two mastectomies, reconstruction hell, and more surgeries.

I could and would conquer the communal dressing room.

The room was about ten by twelve feet, and the girl had positioned herself about three-quarters of the way down the twelve-foot side. Mirrored walls surrounded us, and a continuous narrow bench encircled the room, attached to the wall. A few hooks to hang your garments on were randomly placed, which made positioning yourself a tough task. Braiden carefully hung her selection of blouses across from the girl, and I plopped my bras on the bench.

We exchanged glances with the girl and nodded at the dress she was trying on.

"My ex-fiancé is getting married," she explained. "I'm on my lunch break and don't have much time. I need a killer dress for the wedding."

It is amazing what you learn about a stranger in a short amount of time. Understandably, she needed to look hot, which this dress did, but it was so tight on her voluptuous figure that it made her look desperate.

Braiden leaned in and whispered to me, "You're beautiful." She must have picked up on my anxiety.

As one quickly removes a Band-Aid to avoid the pain, I

tried to strip in one movement. My breasts popped out from my bra and flew everywhere, escaping with lightning speed, as if they had been anticipating the opportune time to bolt for freedom. I was facing the wall, and as I fumbled for them, I only got clumsier. Breasts were falling on the floor, bouncing around like little fleas. The harder I tried to peel the sports bra off, the more my arms and the elastic band of fabric entwined in a tangled web as the fugitive breasts fled.

The poor girl trying on cocktail dresses may not have even noticed the comedy of errors going on. She had on a forest green number that would have made a stick figure look fat. The hem cut her legs off at the worst possible spot, and her arms puffed out of the armholes like marshmallows. She was in her own nightmare.

Any shred of self-esteem I had was gone. Braiden was trying on her newfound treasures, but she had not missed a moment. She and I locked eyes and chuckled as quietly as possible. But Braiden does not do quiet.

With as much grace as I could muster, I gathered the fugitives and slipped them into a sexy black number I was trying on. But now I needed to take that bra off and try another. I refused to traumatize this poor girl any more than she already was by exposing her to my body scars. This meant grasping the breasts with one hand while removing the bra and putting a new one on with the other.

The next one clasped in front. Of course it did. I had finally mastered the back closure and now I was facing a new challenge. It is amazing how much you forget and how hard it is to master bra technique. Pity the poor teenage boy learning this art form with his first girlfriend. I tried to study the mechanism, but I had not brought my glasses, so it was all a blur. Braiden was off in her own world, trying on the latest fashions, and our friend was trying on a bright yellow dress. Clearly this woman needed advice on how to make a man sorry he lost her.

I managed to get the front closure open and put my arms into the straps, but my breasts were nowhere to be found. They had again made their escape and were heading for the hills. Or maybe they were the hills.

My face was beet red, and sweat was on its way. I decided to put the bra on and then try to find my wandering breasts. I figured that since I had mastered opening the closure, it would not be hard to close it and I could do it quickly.

Semi-blind, nerves frayed, sweat pouring, and hands trembling, I found the closure impossible. My face was now the color of the girl's latest red dress calamity.

I summoned Braiden.

"I can't get it either," she mumbled, trying to keep her voice down, which, with Braiden's projection voice, is not possible. We were trying to hold back the giggles, unsuccessfully. I am sure our dressing room companion heard us—how could she not have heard Braiden's squeaks? But she ignored our antics, and I was too flustered to care.

We got the stupid bra closed. I found my breasts on the floor, under some clothes, and slipped them into the bra.

"You need to pull the back of the bra down like this." Braiden tugged it into place. *Thanks, Mom.* Here I am, an accomplished mother of two grown children, unable to put on her own bra. The girl looked over and commented that it looked nice. She must have thought Braiden had a very "challenged" mother.

Three more bras to try on. I was getting more confident and decided that I had humiliated myself to the point that it did not matter what I did or what I exposed or did not expose. I slipped bras on and off and mastered the front closure. The breasts fell in, out, on the floor, on the bench, and I let them go. They wanted to have a mind of their own, and I gave it to them. As with children, you have to let them go in order to keep them.

The three of us, five if you include my breasts, chose a bra. Not the front closure, thank goodness. Our unanimous choice was black, with lace around the top—beautiful and feminine without being overly sexy. I was ready to push myself. I would try on some tops, but I put my sports bra back on for comfort.

"Try these on." Braiden held out the tops she had picked for herself.

I laughed. "Right. Like those are going to fit me."

"Just for style, Mom. So you'll know what shapes look good on you."

She helped me struggle into the clothing.

"Not bad," she whispered. She looked like the cat who ate the canary. She was proud of me. The tops looked good, if I do say so myself, and they were not as tight as I would have thought. I glanced over at our companion, who was about done. She had become quieter as she'd realized she would not accomplish her mission during this lunch hour.

I was feeling confident, even a bit cocky, when Braiden gave my chest a funny sideways stare.

"Mom," she said calmly and as quietly as she could. "You're migrating."

What in the world did that mean? I looked down to see two lumps sitting in the middle of my chest. My little beasts (not a typo) had migrated toward each other.

The poor girl, desperate and about to admit defeat, was trapped in a communal dressing room with two crazy women, in complete hysterics about who knows what. Braiden's big brown eyes were filled with tears, her mouth open wide as she was gasping for air. All that came out were high squeaks.

My breasts had been lonely and decided to meet in the middle. They had been in cahoots to torture me and were getting together to celebrate their victory.

"This is what I had to live with," I whispered to Braiden, who was waving her hands in front of her mouth, still trying to catch her breath. "Now you see why I chose not to have breasts."

This is what I and countless other mastectomy victims have gone through. The breasts have the upper hand. Your choice is to contend with the migrating beasts or Velcro them onto a giant Band-Aid attached to your chest, in either case hoping that they will stay in place. Or you can get one of those ugly Victorianesque torture bras with pockets, hoping they will keep the breasts in place. These were the choices I had consciously and bravely given up more than seventeen years ago. And here I was, back at the beginning. Times had not changed, but I had. I had gone to the mountain and back, feeling like a conqueror and a failure.

Who knows which direction I will take. The clothing line is officially on hold. I am anxious to get back to my art. I do not want to date, but I do want to feel better about my body, and with breasts, I do. Maybe I will get implants. Prostheses are for the birds. But I am terrified of putting something foreign in my body again. What if my body rejects it like it did before? Even worse, what if the symptoms are again so vague that I do not notice my body trying to reject the implants? What if the doctor does a lousy job? Am I up to having surgery every ten years to replace the implants, as doctors recommend? Can I afford the surgery?

I have researched the latest advances in implants, and not a whole lot has changed. A few new products are on the market, but I cannot help being suspicious. My implant had been the latest product, and as soon as I'd finished the painful eight-month reconstruction, the medical community had issued a safety warning for that implant. Would the worry gnaw away at me?

Implants put in under the breast muscle look more natural than those put on top. The problem is that under the muscle requires a more complicated invasive surgery and has the potential to leak into the inner body. On top of the body is a simple surgery, relatively inexpensive, easy to monitor and replace. But to me they look like two half melons stuck on top of your chest. Which is basically what they are.

My chest is riddled with zippers and scar tissue. Why would I want to try implants again, to expose my mind and body to potential trauma? But I want to look good again, and I don't know what to do. Maybe you were expecting that I'd find the answers by the end of this book. Maybe I was expecting that.

Chapter Forty

Full Circle

*S*eptember 11, 2009. I was sitting in my house in Colorado on the overstuffed chair with the poppies that Alan had bought for me, with my pink "hamster" shirt wrapped around me, waiting anxiously by the phone to hear that my house in Bozeman had sold.

I never wanted to sell that house. It was where my family had started a new life after the post-9/11 economic collapse. It was the house where my husband had died, and where Braiden, Chelsea, Ty, and I had altered and resewn our lives to fit without Alan. It was the house where I had become an artist, and where my mission to create an alternative for mastectomy survivors had percolated. I loved this house. I will always love this house.

I had worked hard after Alan died to finish the remodeling and make it a home that he would have been proud of. It was hard to rent it to strangers, and each phone call I got about a repair that needed to be made (and there were many) sent me into a depressed stupor. It was time to move on and sell the house, to let someone else enjoy it. It belonged with someone who would love it, not a bunch of random people looking for a place to stay. I was not going back to Bozeman to live; it was not for me. Not the me I was now.

I asked my tenants to move out. This meant no rental income, and if the house did not sell by the end of summer, I would have to rent it again, which I dreaded.

My property manager (actually my mailman and his wife) and Realtor worked to get the house back to its original beauty. The house was listed in mid-June, and I put it out of my mind.

My agent, Susan, called out of nowhere. I had an inquiry from a young couple who loved the house but could not afford it. They wanted to know if I would consider a much lower offer.

"Please thank them very much," I told her. "Tell them that I can't consider such a low offer, but that I appreciate their love of the house and might consider something in between." Then I put them out of my mind.

We will call them couple number one.

Couple number one presented another offer. The economy was still in a crisis, and Bozeman, which was always at least two years behind the rest of the country, had a much longer way to go to recovery.

"Let's make this offer work," I told Susan.

"All right, I'll do my best," she said, surprised.

They would love the house, I told myself.

We had almost reached an agreement when Susan called.

"You won't believe this," she said. "Another party is interested in the house. After all this time, you have two offers! You're still in negotiations with couple number one, so you can consider another offer."

Couple number two matched couple number one's offer, plus they would pay cash, with a two-week escrow. Even though couple number two wanted to remodel the house (it was perfect; how could they tear it apart?), were from California (a strike against them in Montana), and had a last name that rhymed with "mutt," I accepted their offer. It was questionable if couple number one could qualify for the house, and, I tried to convince myself, it was a business deal.

Couple number two scheduled an inspection. Now tell me, why would anyone expect a house built in 1946 not to have issues? Along with the house's charm comes old.

"You're not going to believe this," Susan said. "I don't know who the inspector was, but he reported that the house 'might' have mold and 'might' have asbestos, and couple number two ran. I couldn't believe that they would run without doing further investigation, but it was their choice. What do you want to do?"

It was back to couple number one to see if they were still interested. They were.

I was in DC again, and my mother had come to spend the week and go to my cousin's daughter's wedding in New York. It had been a stressful week of traveling with family and the typical multigenerational drama. My blood pressure needed a break.

"You're not going to believe this."

Susan and I were getting used to this start in our conversations.

Another couple was making an offer. This was crazy. The market was terrible, and here I was, with three couples interested in my house. Had I priced it too low, or did others see what a special house it was?

"Haven't had this much action in years," Susan exclaimed. "Let me see what I can do."

"When this house finally closes," I told Susan, "I'm going to eat ice cream all day long."

It had been a very long week. Ben and I took my mother to the Baltimore airport, and as we were walking through the terminal, Susan called. She had told couple number three that we had multiple offers, and that if they wanted to make an offer, it had better be good. The cell phone reception was lousy, so I lost the connection before she could finish.

I could call Susan back later. I needed to get my mother to the airport gate. At security, I showed the TSA agent the pass I'd gotten to go through with her to security, but he just smirked when he looked at it. He was not about to let me go through. My mother's name had been put on it by mistake, not mine. As Ben and I were running back to the ticket counter, the phone rang again. This time Susan was able to get through to me that the couple had offered full price. Full price! I quickly accepted couple number three's offer, and poor couple number one lost again.

Ben was able to get the ticket agent to give me a new pass with my name on it. We ran back to the same TSA agent, and I shoved the pass in his face, then ran to catch up to my mother, who was just getting through security. On our way out of the airport, Susan called yet again. "We need to sign the papers now!" she said. "This is a deal we can't lose. Can you get to a fax or email?"

Oddly, the airport had no business center for sending and receiving faxes and emails. So Ben and I stopped at a Kinko's on the way home. I was able to receive, copy, sign, and fax acceptance of the full price offer.

I couldn't believe this. I felt exonerated. The house was worth what I thought it was. Alan would have been proud; I had done a good job. I knew that the couple would find lots of issues with the inspection, but full price gave me lots of wiggle room to negotiate. I could almost taste the ice cream. It seemed too good to be true.

Which of course meant that it was.

The next day, Susan called again.

One "You're not going to believe this" later and she'd explained that the wife in couple number three had recently been diagnosed with breast cancer. "She was just informed that she has been accepted into an experimental program in Salt Lake City. Rightfully so, they do not feel that they could handle a new house and the medical treatment at the same time."

My heart went out to them. How random is it that she would be dealing with breast cancer? I wanted to let these strangers to know how much I felt for them and how I wanted to help them in any way I could. But all I could do was say how sorry I was and let them go.

"Is couple number one still around?"

"Don't know, but I'll sure find out." I think Susan was having the time of her life.

Was couple number one still around? Much to my surprise, yes. I hoped it was meant to be. The price was not the best, but it could work. I would make it work. I loved this house more than any other. It embodied who I was, and it was going to be so hard to let it go, but at least it would be in good hands. Sweet couple number one. They had hung in there, and we agreed on the terms.

Next hurdle was the home inspection. We requested a copy of the original inspection report from couple number two.

"The inspector must have had nothing else to do when he did this," Susan reported. "His final report was fifty-seven pages long! I've never seen such a report."

It apparently included such details as "the righthand corner of the left wall on the northeast, which is the corner of the right wall on the north side, has a small one-inch crack in it."

"This is the craziest report I've ever seen," she exclaimed, "No wonder couple number two ran. I hope I never have to deal with that inspector again."

We gave the report to couple number one and anxiously waited. There were no indications that a couple number four was about to appear. I wanted this deal to work.

Couple number one brought their own inspector to the house. No signs of asbestos or mold. At least we were over that hurdle. The house did have some other issues, so now I waited for couple number one to tell me what repairs they wanted.

They asked for reasonable repairs, and I was happy to comply. There was another tense moment when their agent would not accept the wording of the repairs from the plumber, even though the inspector said it was repaired. We were all so frustrated and tense; the sale was about to fall through because of the direction the basement showerhead turned.

But then couple number one accepted the repairs, and it was on to the final escrow.

On Friday, September 11, 2009, at 11:02 A.M., I was back in Colorado, in my poppy chair.

The phone rang. It was Susan. "It's time to have ice cream."

Of all days for it to close—September 11, the start of my journey, starting with the 9/11 tragedy and Alan losing his job. I sank further into the womb of my poppy chair, gazing out the window at the Rockies. I often saw deer wandering across my yard, and I hoped that I would see one today.

After what seemed like ages, I got up, grabbed a spoon and the carton of ice cream, and returned to my chair.

I sank into it as far as I could.

Tears mixed in with chocolate chip vanilla bean. The house was gone. Alan was gone. Our dream of a simple life in a mountain town was gone. My crusade to liberate women from breasts was gone.

I dialed Jamie's number, composing my thoughts.

But then all the words I had planned to say seemed irrelevant. I took a deep breath, closed my eyes, and, with a slight grin, whispered:

"Still alive."

Acknowledgments

When I told my family and friends that my book was going to be published, the unanimous response was,

"You wrote a book?"

It was the last thing anyone, including myself, thought I would do.

With that in mind, I would like to first acknowledge "The Michaels," who got me into this. Michael Sussman, my DC landlord and friend, the consummate "connector," who introduced me to my publisher and mentor, Michael Vezo. From a casual meeting, mentioning under my breath that I had scribbled a book, to actually publishing a book has been one of the most incredible experiences I have ever had. Michael V. taught me a valuable lesson in life, using his words:

"Never say no to an opportunity."

Michael V. introduced me to Melanie Mallon, my editor. With the gentleness and firmness of a parent, she took a self-proclaimed nonwriter and transformed me into a person who now loves the written word. She is truly a miracle worker.

Michael V. also introduced me to Chris Flynn, who, with much patience and talent, helped to create the book cover.

Acknowledgments

My precious family (in order of appearance) has been essential in writing this story. My parents, Sid and Nee, gave me the confidence to do anything and the opportunity to accomplish it. Jamie, Lauren, Alan, Karren, Brighton, Chelsea, Ty, Fred, and Andrew not only encouraged, supported, and loved me in my life and in this process, but they have been my cheering squad and invaluable critics. They pushed me to dig deep, beyond my limits, and challenged me not to accept "good enough." They taught me to be honest, give up control, and let it happen. Plus, they gave me great material to write about.

Finally, my family of friends, you know who you are (yes, Keitho), has stuck with me through the good, the bad, and the unexpected. Their friendship and support have given me the confidence to pursue my obsessions and helped me to believe that I am okay.

Thank you all.

CPSIA information can be obtained at www.ICGtesting.com
Printed in the USA
LVOW040659200113

316386LV00001B/2/P

9 781938 620010